Women and Health
Cultural and Social Perspectives

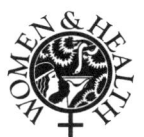

Modern Mothers
in the Heartland

Gender, Health, and Progress in Illinois, 1900–1930

Lynne Curry

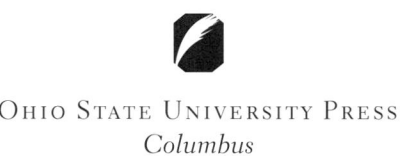

OHIO STATE UNIVERSITY PRESS

Columbus

Library of Congress Cataloging-in-Publication Data

Curry, Lynne.
Modern mothers in the heartland : gender, health, and progress in Illinois,
1990–1930 / Lynne Curry.
p.   cm. — (Women and health)
Includes bibliographical references and index.
ISBN 0-8142-0830-4 (cloth : alk. paper) — ISBN 0-8142-5032-7 (pbk. : alk. paper)
1. Health promotion — Illinois.   2. Health education of women — Illinois.   3. Women
health reformers — Illinois.   4. Maternal and infant welfare — Illinois.   I. Title.
II. Series: Women & health (Columbus, Ohio)
RA447.I3C87   1999
613'.082'09773 — dc21   99-27611
CIP

Text and cover design by Gary Gore.
Type set in Electra by Graphic Composition, Inc.
Printed by Sheridan Books.

9 8 7 6 5 4 3 2 1

To the memory of my mother and father

CONTENTS

ACKNOWLEDGMENTS

It was my great good fortune to enjoy the guidance of a number of generous scholars, and the support of many helpful peers, as I navigated my work through its various phases from graduate seminar paper to doctoral dissertation to published monograph. My sincere appreciation goes to the series editors, Rima D. Apple and Janet Golden, for providing me with the opportunity to make my book a part of their exciting project. I especially wish to thank Rima Apple for her insightful suggestions and steady encouragement as the manuscript slowly but surely took on its final form.

Over the past eight years Sonya Michel has shared with me her vast knowledge of the historiography of women and gender as well as her critical insights into Progressive Era maternalist politics. I have grown professionally under her sound guidance as well. Leslie J. Reagan was especially generous with both her limited time and her seemingly unlimited expertise as she aided and advised my earliest explorations into the history of public health and medicine in the United States. Her own excellent scholarship remains a model that I can only hope to emulate. James R. Barrett and Mark Leff conducted rigorous seminars in which I honed my skills in the historian's crafts of research and writing; I still count my fellow graduate students in those seminars among the most exacting critics of my work. This book is also the product of invaluable comments and critiques provided at different stages in its development by Barbara Hobson, John Hoffman, Fred Jaher, Joan Jensen, Stacey Robertson, Chris Waldrep, participants in the Feminist Scholarship Series at the University of Illinois at Urbana-Champaign, and the anonymous reviewers for the Ohio State University Press. Through her efficient professionalism and good humor Charlotte Dihoff has done much to help assuage the anxieties of the publication process. Any errors, however, remain my own responsibility.

My research excursions have been greatly assisted by the efforts of librarians and archivists too numerous to mention individually. I owe a debt of appreciation to the library staffs at the University of Illinois and Eastern Illinois University for their help in locating and obtaining archival records,

xACKNOWLEDGMENTS

government documents, and a number of rather ephemeral publications over the years. I have also received indispensable assistance from personnel at the Illinois Historical Survey, the Chicago Historical Society, the Midwest Women's History Collection at the University of Illinois at Chicago, the Illinois State Archives, the Illinois State Library, the Rural Oral History Project at the University of Illinois at Springfield, and several local and county historical collections. Funding from the University of Illinois in the form of a fellowship, a research assistantship, and a dissertation research grant allowed me to complete the doctoral dissertation from which this book developed.

I have learned that one grows a good deal, both personally and professionally, from endeavors such as this. A kindly word of encouragement from Linda Kerber at the very beginning of my academic career helped convince me I was on the right track. The supportive community created by the History Women's Caucus at the University of Illinois reminded me at several critical junctures that the project I had undertaken was indeed worthwhile. Special acknowledgment goes to my treasured colleagues in the History Department at Eastern Illinois University from whom I continue to learn much about being a historian. Over the years the interest in my work shown by numerous family members extending over the miles from Martinez, California, to Fayette, Alabama, has meant a great deal to this transplant to the Midwest. I wish to thank especially Michele Watts, James Lewanski, Margaret Vinnedge, and Judy Shewry. Finally, but by no means least importantly, I owe my deepest debt of gratitude to Brandon, Ian, and Samuel Curry who remain my most important sources of inspiration.

INTRODUCTION

Whatever your definition of progress may be,
health is an essential factor.

In 1920 Caroline Hedger, a Chicago physician well acquainted with public health conditions in that midwestern industrial city, traveled south to the rural "downstate" region of Illinois in order to address the Women's Department of the Farmers' Institute. The topic of Hedger's presentation was, "The Relation of Health to Progress."[1] Improving physical well-being in Illinois — and in particular, safeguarding the health of that state's youngest citizens and the mothers who bore and raised them — stood at the very center of the vision of social progress built by reformers like Hedger during the first two decades of the twentieth century. A broad coalition of public health practitioners, social welfare advocates, and women's rights supporters argued that a sound and democratic future depended upon mothers' ability to produce and maintain a robust citizenry. Like their counterparts elsewhere in the nation, health reformers in Illinois linked the latest scientific advances in the germ theory together with their own drive to bring social progress to their state, constructing a distinctive and dynamic ideology that historian Nancy Tomes has labeled "hygienic modernism."[2] Modern mothers, this credo insisted, need not passively accept ill health and untimely death as God's mysterious will or the work of Divine Providence. Instead, women could exert substantial control over their own physical states as well as those of future generations by conscientiously following the precepts of preventive health and household hygiene.

Battling what they saw as a self-defeating propensity for "superstition" and "fatalism" regarding illness and untimely death among too many residents of their state, Illinois reformers attempted to inculcate among urban and rural mothers alike a new, higher standard for defining what it meant to be "in good health." Representatives of local women's clubs, philanthropic agencies, agricultural extension services, and public health departments

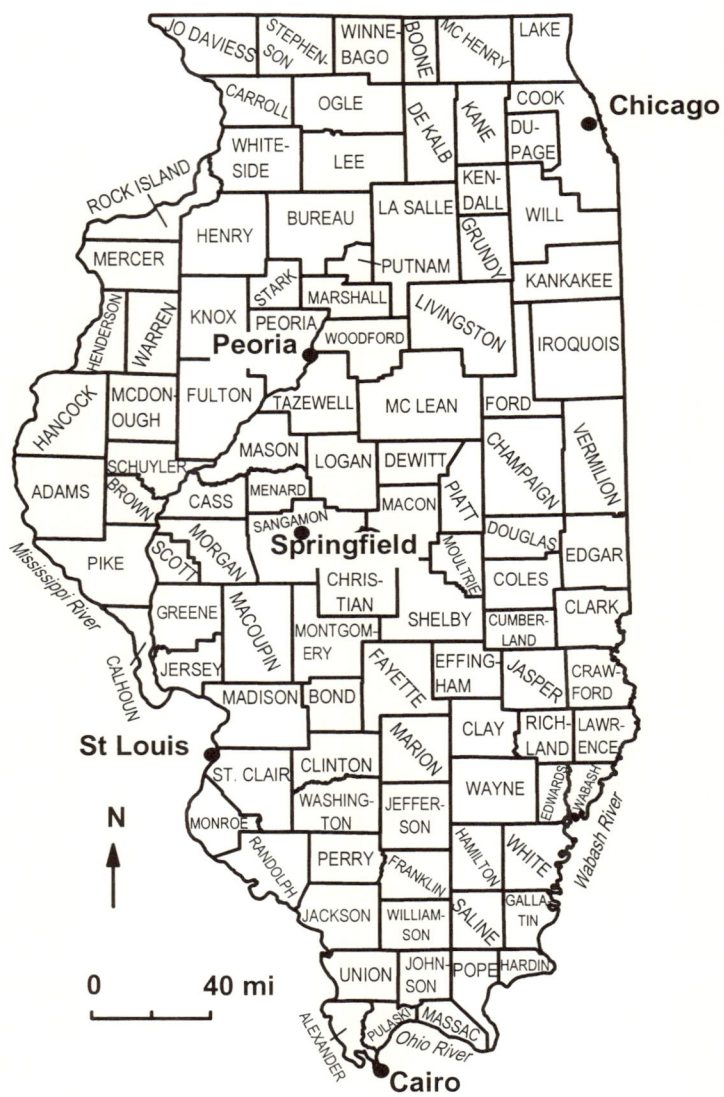

carried the modernization-through-better-hygiene message throughout the state, utilizing methods as diverse as the mass distribution of child care pamphlets, domestic sanitation lessons for farm wives, English language classes imparting a preventive health vocabulary to immigrant mothers, and "better baby" contests demonstrating infant hygiene at agricultural fairs. Integrally tied to a larger reform agenda that encompassed Americanizing Chicago's immigrants and uplifting the agrarian population, preventive health campaigns recruited mothers from cities, small towns, and rural villages, welding them into a sizable grassroots maternal force whose ultimate goal was no less ambitious than the modernization of America's heartland. The combination of pragmatic lessons in preventing the onset of illness and the lofty imagery of midwestern modernity brought an unprecedented vitality to the Illinois health reform movement, establishing a prominent place for that state in the vanguard of progressive reform.[3]

The special attentions Illinois health reformers paid to the well-being of their state's youngest and most vulnerable residents reflected the overriding concern with child welfare that marked Progressive Era social movements in the United States. As the accurate and systematic recording of births and deaths became more widespread, newly available statistics revealed that childhood mortality rates had stayed shockingly high despite notable decreases in the overall death rate. Further, such revelations came to light within an ideological climate that stressed efficiency and rationality as hallmarks of social progress. In an advanced nation such as the United States, the persistence of ill health and high death rates among future citizens and workers seemed not only distressingly counterproductive but even somewhat barbaric, a throwback to an earlier, less enlightened time. Social reformers, child welfare advocates, and public health officials were allied in the view that, for the good of the nation, childhood death could no longer be regarded as a private family tragedy but instead must be recognized as a shared societal problem demanding the public's foremost attention. Appreciating the complex causes underlying many childhood illnesses, they argued for wide-ranging and coordinated attacks across economic, social, and political fronts. In 1907, the campaign against early death gained a national forum when child welfare advocates founded the American Association for Study and Prevention of Infant Mortality (AASPIM).[4]

For health reformers in Illinois, the untimely deaths of babies and young children seemed all the more distressing because they knew many of these tragedies could be prevented. The medical paradigm informing health reform efforts had changed significantly in recent decades. Advances in the new science of bacteriology had made it possible to identify the environmental germs responsible for causing a number of ailments all too familiar to both urban and rural midwesterners, including typhoid fever, dysentery, and many of the diarrheal diseases of childhood. With these discoveries came new hope that such devastating afflictions could be brought under control through the widespread and systematic practice of basic prophylactic measures.

Historians of medicine note a critical shift in public health strategies at this time, as "New Public Health" advocates turned their attentions away from the large-scale engineering of the urban environment and concentrated instead on changing the human behaviors now understood to contribute significantly to the spread of disease. While nineteenth-century public health improvement efforts had centered primarily on periodic — and often devastating — visitations of epidemic diseases to local communities, more recent discoveries in bacteriology had made it apparent that the true menace to well-being did not always attack the community from the outside but instead lurked completely unnoticed within the seemingly benign everyday milieu of the household and neighborhood. Women continued to deliver their babies assisted by untrained midwives, helpful neighbors, and even medical doctors who remained largely ignorant of the hazards of infection posed by their own unwashed hands and unsterilized implements. Naive mothers fed their babies unpasteurized milk in unsterilized bottles and put their little ones down to sleep on bedding infested with microscopic germs.[5]

Thus, preventive health reformers extolled the mundane actions mothers performed within their own households such as frequent hand-washing, boiling the family drinking water, and screening nursery windows to keep out disease-carrying flies not merely as feminine domestic virtues but as vital measures for safeguarding the nation's future strength, serious work that would enable a modern nation to grow and to thrive. Mothers' routine private duties in providing preventive health care thereby took on an unparalleled public significance. While a belief in women's special obligations for maintaining cleanliness and order had informed health reform efforts in earlier decades, by 1900 such female moral imperatives had secured a solid scientific rationale in the germ theory.

Gender figured prominently in the health campaigns launched in the early twentieth century. Historically, care of the sick and injured had formed an integral part of the domestic economy for which generations of wives and mothers assumed responsibility.[6] Rural communities isolated from the services of medical professionals depended heavily upon the healing skills of local women. Drawing upon a vast store of information gleaned from family custom, folk wisdom, and popular advice manuals, midwestern mothers had doctored their little ones through the various ailments of childhood and counseled female kin and neighbors during the stages of pregnancy and new motherhood.

In the mid-nineteenth century, such pragmatic necessities became sentimentalized in popular Victorian tributes to the healing properties of maternal love, a special set of virtues instinctive to the female sex. But by the century's end, the increasingly widespread awareness of the germ theory brought an unprecedented urgency to a mother's nurturing duties; new and alarming information about microscopic dangers in the environment demanded that every mother keep up to date on the latest methods for safeguarding the health of her household. Modern motherhood became an exacting occupation, a quasi-scientific vocation requiring women to obtain advanced education and specialized training. "The owner of a motor car is not willing to entrust his machine to a novice," Minnie Ahrens of the Infant Welfare Society of Chicago offered in analogy in 1915. "The mechanism of a baby, which is far more delicate and intricate than that of a motor car and there is the disadvantage that broken parts cannot be replaced, is often entrusted to a novice in Motherhood." In a society undergoing rapid transformation by the forces of industrialization, urbanization, and modernization the work of mothering had become far too complex to be entrusted to maternal instinct alone. The new field of home economics being pioneered by Isabel Bevier at the University of Illinois and her female colleagues at college campuses elsewhere would help to meet the heartland's need for a modern, scientific approach to motherhood.[7]

But, if women represented the primary objects of health reform in this era, they could also be counted among its most active agents. A "maternalist" ideology deeply rooted in long-standing cultural traditions that assumed a female prerogative in matters of children's welfare served as an entering wedge for women's participation in public-sphere campaigns for social reform.[8] Like their counterparts in other states, a significant number of educated and socially prominent women in Illinois joined a range of progressive reform movements with enthusiasm, giving special attention to causes promoting the well-being of mothers and children. Although the Illinois State Board of Health had been established in 1877, its operations were primarily confined to licensing medical practitioners. Underfinanced and unfavored by the state legislature in Springfield, the state's public health infrastructure remained scant well into the twentieth century.[9] Activities designed to enlighten the general public on the modern precepts of preventive health and hygiene therefore relied heavily on support from volunteers in local communities. Elite women in the Chicago Woman's Club, for example, initiated, financed, and supported many of that city's maternal and child health programs, while well-to-do farm women downstate organized health instruction programs through the Women's Department of the Illinois Farmers' Institute. Female volunteers staffed the front lines of health reform as they

erected exhibits at agricultural fairs, delivered lectures at summer Chautau-
quas, and narrated magic lantern shows in local movie houses. Women in
both urban and rural regions of Illinois also participated in a lively discourse
on the importance of good health in a modern society carried out within the
pages of farm journals and popular women's magazines.

The unprecedented public significance that Illinois progressives attached to women's traditional health care duties created a new role for
women in civic affairs. Shut out from mainstream political structures in their
state, the women activists who provided both financial backing and volunteer support to numerous public health and social welfare campaigns in Illinois succeeded in building what historian Kathleen D. McCarthy has
described as "parallel power structures" during the decades prior to the en-
actment of women's suffrage. Members of the elite Chicago Woman's Club,
a steady supporter of health reform campaigns in that city, viewed their organization as "a finely equipped training school, wherein one thousand
thinking women absorb the knowledge which is power — power in the civic
life of Chicago."[10] The founding of the Children's Bureau within the United
States Department of Labor in 1912 marked both a watershed in maternalist
health care advocacy in the United States and an unprecedented place for
women in government service. The Bureau's first chief, Chicago settlement
house worker and social welfare activist Julia Lathrop, made the reduction
of infant mortality the new agency's top priority. By the 1910s, the vigorous
endeavors of a number of prominent social welfare institutions in Chicago —
most notably Hull House under the direction of its visionary cofounder, Jane
Addams — had transformed that city into an important training ground for
female leadership in child health and welfare campaigns at the national
level. With Lathrop's appointment to the Children's Bureau, Chicago became a major node in the dynamic network of female reformers that now
crisscrossed the nation.[11]

Recently, scholars have begun to call for broader conceptual frame-
works in order to capture the full complexity of health and social welfare
movements in the United States. To date, most historians heeding this call
have focused on developments on the national scene.[12] By contrast, this
study of Illinois in the first decades of the twentieth century examines the
historical intersections of progressivism, maternalism, and health reform as
they merged into an energetic and diverse social reform movement in one
state during a period that witnessed profound changes in the formulation of
health care policies and the delivery of health care services. In shifting the

focus of historical inquiry away from national policies, institutions, and actors, and toward the state and local levels, a more intricate picture emerges of the interplay among multiple factors including gender, ethnicity, class, and regional distinctiveness as they shaped and reshaped Progressive Era reform. In addition, a focus on Illinois allows us to discern shades of difference among health reform campaigns taking place in the burgeoning industrial metropolis of Chicago and the small towns and rural villages of downstate communities.

As a group, Illinois health reform activists differed considerably in their training, experience, and the specific strategies they chose to endorse. Private charitable organizations, elite urban women's clubs, agricultural extension services, and public health bodies all lent crucial human and financial resources to the cause. Despite their varying backgrounds, however, all participants could agree that the widespread dissemination of preventive health and hygiene information represented a vital means for advancing social progress in the state. Initially at least, Illinois reformers were also united by a conviction that because the future belonged to the young, all of the state's residents shared a special, intrinsic interest in safeguarding the health of mothers and children.

Health reform in the period from 1900 to 1930 developed within a larger context of rapid and often unsettling change. Like other midwestern states, Illinois experienced major transformations in its demographic composition in this period. In 1900, the urban and rural populations in the state were roughly equivalent. By 1920, however, a two-to-one majority lived in towns and cities; and by 1930, nearly three out of four of that state's residents were urban dwellers. Further, many of these profound changes in the social landscape did not occur evenly. Illinois extends southward from its border with Wisconsin for approximately four hundred miles, a distance that creates notable geographical and climatological differences within the boundaries of the state. The northern tip rests on the same latitude as the city of Boston, Massachusetts, while its southern end parallels Richmond, Virginia. Political, economic, and cultural variations between the state's extreme northern and southern regions had significant consequences for both the state of peoples' health and the development of campaigns for reform. By 1900 northern Illinois, heavily influenced by the population size, industrial might, and political dominance of Chicago, shared a variety of characteristics in common with the nation's industrialized and urbanized northeast, while the southern portion of Illinois in many respects bore a much closer resemblance to the rural South.[13] As late as 1930, disparities in public health conditions between the state's northern and southern regions remained very much in evidence.

Perhaps inescapably, health reformers throughout Illinois fashioned their campaigns from the convictions of their own socioeconomic class. Germs, as public health practitioners were fond of pointing out, respected no social or economic boundaries, and illness could be passed (apparently unilaterally) from the poor to the wealthy, from the country to the city, from immigrants to the native-born. Arguably, then, it was a simple matter of bourgeois self-interest that the masses with whom they shared public spaces be taught basic scientific principles of preventive health and hygiene. But Progressive Era health reform was about more than shielding the middle classes from disease. Bound to a much grander vision of modernization, re-formers also intended their preventive health campaigns to transmit middle-class values using the daily household work performed by mothers as the engine of change. By the late nineteenth century a clean home, healthy children, and orderly neighborhood had come to serve as symbols of Ameri-can middle-class culture, signposts by which urban, native-born, and afflu-ent families could distinguish themselves from their rural, foreign-born, and poorer neighbors.[14]

Progressives imagined the modern American their reforms would help to create as an exceptionally robust and vigorous individual who naturally preferred to live in an updated, sanitized home situated on a clean, orderly street. Thus, preventive health and hygiene education programs also served as models delineating what the attributes of a modern American identity should be. Further, educational activities stressing personal and household hygiene offered some exceedingly pragmatic lessons in how one could *be-come* both modern and American. Chicago-based health reformers, firmly rooted in the urban middle-classes themselves, insisted that training foreign-born mothers in the health habits already practiced by native-born women would accelerate the process of acculturation in ethnic communities. Like-wise, university-trained agricultural extension agents working in downstate farming communities sought to remove the dirt and drudgery from rural motherhood in order to make it more closely resemble the bourgeois ideal posited for city mothers, promoting what historian Mary Neth has called "middle-class modernity" as the appropriate model to be emulated by the country mothers they hoped to engage in the cause.[15] Progressive Era health reformers adhered to a core belief that social progress could be realized by promoting a higher standard of health and hygiene among those currently living outside the boundaries of the urban, native-born middle class. Their faith in the transformative power of education separated progressive health reformers from the strictest eugenicists among their contemporaries for whom preventive health and hygiene campaigns merely represented a misguided attempt to sustain the inferior and the weak.[16]

It would be a mistake, however, to dismiss health reform in the early twentieth century as nothing more than a form of social control by which one class sought to dominate another. First, as historians of maternalist politics in this era have pointed out, elite women who joined campaigns to combat infection following childbirth and the loss of infants due to diarrheal diseases were not themselves entirely liberated from these all-too-common hazards of early twentieth-century life. For the most political among maternalists, persistently high rates of adult female death from childbirth-related causes represented graphic evidence that women had not received their proper share of attention from the state.[17] Second, a closer look at activities taking place at the local level in Illinois allows us to see more clearly the *interactive* nature of reform as actors on various tiers — policymakers at public and private agencies, mothers in cities and rural areas, and the scores of women volunteers who worked between them — all made identifiable contributions to the cause. Third, a crude social control analysis obscures the fact that health reform held tangible rewards for people among whom high rates of disease and death still lingered like a pernicious shadow. In the absence of infection-fighting drugs, preventive health and hygiene education constituted the best weapon available in the Progressive Era war against disease. As historians Neil N. Cowan and Ruth Schwartz Cowan point out, immigrants from southern and eastern Europe gained more potent weapons against childhood disease in their first twenty years in America than tradition had offered them over two millennia.[18] High attendance numbers regularly recorded at various health education events in both rural and urban venues across the state indicate that the message of modernization through better health was one a great many Illinois residents were ready to hear.

Finally, including a grassroots perspective in the examination of progressive health reform illuminates the movement's underlying promises about social mobility in America.[19] For the immigrant mother raising her children in the tenements of Chicago, the incorporation of modern American-style practices into her existing repertoire of folk medicine and child care traditions could serve as a sort of badge verifying to those both inside and outside her community that she had successfully adapted to her new home. Editors of foreign-language newspapers in Chicago urged their female readers to attend and listen attentively to public health lectures so their domestic hygiene habits would not serve as an embarrassment to the immigrant community. In America, "a woman must be enlightened in the duties required or she will not be able to fill that high position of home-maker and mother," asserted the Polish National Alliance through its Chicago-based newspaper, the *Dziennik Zwiazkowy*.[20] Through her participation in preventive health education programs the immigrant mother learned that American mothers gave birth and raised their children in comfort and cleanliness, and as an American-in-the-making such high standards were also hers to enjoy.

Similarly, middle-class activists in segregated Chicago's black public health movement started from an underlying assumption that a clean home, healthy children, and sanitary surroundings connoted a desirable image of social respectability, thereby serving as a means of elevating the entire African American community. Black activists in Chicago, for example, promoted periodic neighborhood cleanup campaigns during "Negro Health Week" as important vehicles for racial uplift.[21] In the downstate region of Illinois, the relatively affluent farm women who became major supporters of public health campaigns in the countryside quite self-consciously tied the goal of rural health reform to their own emerging identity as members of the middle class.

Progressive preventive health campaigns developed first in Chicago, where notoriously poor conditions since the days of earliest white settlement rendered endemic public health problems easily identifiable. As a frontier town Chicago had experienced its first major encounter with deadly cholera in 1832, and within two years civic leaders launched a board of health for the express purpose of responding to the threat posed by this dreaded disease. After the Civil War the city underwent a period of precipitous growth and the resultant overcrowded housing, garbage collection problems, and chronically smoke-filled air all contributed to a public health picture that was dismal indeed. Many of Chicago's burgeoning new industries dumped their waste products directly into the Chicago River, producing an indescribable stench and actually rendering the river solid at times.[22]

But, if Chicago had earned a reputation as an infamously unhealthy place in the 1800s, by century's end it had also emerged as a major center for progressive reform. An energetic network of public health practitioners, social welfare advocates, and maternalist activists from both the private and public sectors mobilized to improve the state of Chicagoans' health. Neighborhood studies using the latest techniques in social science uncovered exceptionally high rates of maternal and infant mortality among the city's immigrant communities. In the period from 1880 to 1910, Chicago saw its foreign-born population increase by more than one-half million, and the conspicuous presence of so many new arrivals from peasant backgrounds prompted considerable concern for the apparent difficulties of assimilating Old Country people into a modern industrial metropolis. Although between 1890 and 1924 the percentage of immigrants barred from entry into the United States because of poor health never exceeded 3 percent each year, many native-born reformers regarded high rates of illness and death in Chicago as problems being imported into the city rather than the result of existing conditions these new residents encountered upon their arrival. Lamentably, this perspective led many Chicago health reformers to pay woefully inadequate attention to the equally pressing public health needs of the thousands of African Americans who were also migrating to the city in this period.

Because they tended to associate poor public health practices with the foreign-born streaming into Chicago's tenement blocks, Illinois health reformers rather belatedly acknowledged that primitive sanitary conditions and a shocking ignorance of proper hygiene practices also prevailed throughout many of the state's rural communities, where residents were overwhelmingly native-born. The incidence of typhoid fever, tuberculosis, and maternal and child deaths in a number of downstate counties was as high as that found in the poorest, most overcrowded tenement districts of Chicago.[23] During its frontier period, dating from approximately 1815 to 1850, Illinois had gained a nefarious reputation as a virtual graveyard for white settlers venturing out to the midwestern prairies from the northeastern and Middle Atlantic states. Although the state did not keep mortality statistics systematically before 1880, there is ample anecdotal evidence from homesteaders themselves attesting to the prevalence of sickness, especially the deadly "bilious" fevers brought on by water-borne diseases such as cholera and typhoid, that plagued the flood-prone region. Malaria, for example, wiped out fully 80 percent of the population of one Illinois county in the 1820s. "Your father had a shake of the ague," Mrs. Tilson of Pike County related in an 1821 letter. "He shuk the hull cabin."[24]

Thus, the persistence of ill health and untimely death in numerous rural counties seemed to many health reformers a regression to these earlier, less enlightened times. "Just across the boundary line from Chicago," Harriet Fulmer of the Illinois State Association for the Prevention of Tuberculosis declared of rural Cook County in 1919, "is a territory covering six hundred square miles, populated by a quarter of a million people, who need as much instruction as the most benighted region of the United States, as far as

matters of health are concerned."[25] Under the illumination of the germ theory, comfortable features of rural midwestern life such as dairy barns, milk
houses, and one-room school buildings now looked more like pernicious
lairs harboring contagious illness. The issue of poor health in the country
was catapulted into the spotlight during the First World War when a higher
percentage of draftees from Illinois farms than from its cities were rejected
as physically unfit for service; medical examiners found malnutrition and
tuberculosis to be surprisingly common among rural recruits.[26]

Ignoring significant socioeconomic differences among the state's rural
population itself, urban-based reformers offered up the poor health conditions they discovered in the countryside as alarming evidence of a more gen-
eralized deterioration afflicting agrarian life. Such alarmist rhetoric to the
contrary, health conditions in the country had not actually become worse,
of course; rural areas had simply failed to keep up with the modern sanitary
advances that by 1900 had already brought notable improvements to Chicago and its environs. Nevertheless, health hazards once considered a routine part of midwestern rural life were recast by health reformers into
alarming social problems requiring immediate remediation.[27] While they often portrayed mothers and babies as the primary victims of unsanitary conditions in the country, health reformers also assigned to farm women a good
deal of responsibility for safeguarding the quality of agrarian life. Unlike Chicago, the downstate region lacked an organized network of middle-class and
elite women activists to champion the special health needs of women and
children. Home economists, public health officials, and agricultural extension agents therefore carved out a central place for farm women in preventive health education campaigns, actively encouraging local female
leadership as part of a larger strategy to modernize rural conditions.[28]

The issue of maternal and child health received a major boost during
the First World War when the Woman's Committee of the Illinois Council
of Defense spearheaded a statewide drive to conserve the health of mothers
and children as an emergency "war measure." Thousands of women throughout the state participated in these home-front activities. While the wartime
maternal and infant health campaign in Illinois reflected some of the most
regrettably conformist and repressive aspects of the American scene in this
period, the movement's widespread popularity — as well as its leaders' unmistakable flair for the dramatic — accentuated the inherent public value of
mothers' special contributions to the national interest. But such unprecedented publicity for the social value of motherhood came at a political price.
In thrusting once sacrosanct maternal responsibilities beyond Victorian sen-

timent and into the arena of public policy-making, health reformers also unwittingly exposed motherly duties to the harsher political realities of dissension, divisiveness, and debate.

In the postwar years, the imprecise boundaries between the public and private spheres that had characterized the development of preventive health care in the Progressive Era created serious political tensions in the state. By the early 1920s, a struggle had ensued to stake out new parameters for the delivery of health care education and services, programs which in Illinois had developed largely outside the offices of doctors in private practice.[29] Due in large part to progressives' own relentless assertion that a healthy citizenry was indispensable to a modern society, preventive health care had become too crucial a matter to be entrusted to the inexpert hands of the lay practitioner.

In 1923, a contentious public policy debate erupted when a major maternalist effort, spearheaded by the Illinois League of Women Voters and supported by the Illinois State Department of Public Health, set out to convince the state's General Assembly to implement the Sheppard-Towner Act in Illinois. Enacted by Congress in 1921, Sheppard-Towner granted federal funds on a state-matching basis for maternal and child health programs. Supporters in Illinois saw this legislation as an unprecedented opportunity to bolster their own long-standing efforts in preventive health and hygiene education. Their campaign, however, was challenged in Springfield by an alliance of business and medical leaders alarmed that Illinois appeared to be headed down a slippery slope toward "state medicine." For the act's opponents, Sheppard-Towner represented an ominous harbinger of the unwelcome encroachment of government intrusion into private life. In an age of scientific motherhood and the right to vote, maternalists entered into the rough-and-tumble of Illinois politics not as mothers with an unassailable moral mission but rather as one special interest among many competing for legislators' attention. Ultimately, Illinois lost the opportunity to enhance its own meager public health apparatus by becoming one of only three states (including Massachusetts and Connecticut) that did not participate in the Sheppard-Towner Act.

Throughout the 1920s in Illinois, sweeping campaigns to advance social welfare by improving the public's physical well-being lost momentum as reformers failed to translate the popularity of preventive health and hygiene programs into solid grassroots political support for the expansion of state-sponsored health services. Further, the defeat of Sheppard-Towner in Illinois presaged a nationwide reaction against greater state responsibility in matters of maternal and child health and welfare in this period. Following their victory in 1923, Illinois physicians joined with their politically ascendent colleagues in the American Medical Association (headquartered in Chicago) to defeat the act on the national level. The Illinois State Medical Society, in fact, moved to the forefront of the national campaign that led to Sheppard-Towner's ultimate demise in 1929. Ironically, then, Illinois managed to retain its position on the cutting edge of health reform well into the 1920s by also leading the decade's backlash against the further expansion of the welfare state.

The controversy over federal funding for preventive health programs in Illinois illustrates with particular clarity a distinctive shift toward the private commodification of health care in the 1920s. Through the decade, physicians in the Illinois State Medical Society railed against the overuse and "abuse" of free and low-cost medical services in Chicago — oddly enough, by the very people whose own expectations for a healthier life progressives had worked so hard to raise. "There is no more reason why people should have free medical service," Dr. Emmet Keating declared before the Chicago Physicians' Fellowship Club in 1927, "than there is that they should have free coal, free rent, free gasoline or any other of the necessities or luxuries of life."[30] The Progressive Era's resounding claim that better health represented the foundation of social advancement had been largely supplanted by a privatized orientation toward the delivery of health care goods and services. Public health practitioners, social workers, and neighborhood infant welfare stations all came under criticism from physicians and business leaders for derailing mothers and children away from private doctors' offices.

But, if preventive health care was moving out of the sphere of social reform and into the marketplace, it is also clear that the goal of modernity through better health had yet to be realized by the poorest and most remote residents of the state. Rates of mortality due to tuberculosis, typhoid fever, and infant diarrheal diseases, for example, remained relatively high in the southernmost counties of the state, even to the end of the decade. While real improvements in the population's health did indeed come to Illinois, they were reached only unevenly at best. In the first decades of the twentieth century, the preventive health and hygiene movement offered Illinois mothers a vision of modernity built upon a new and higher standard of health for themselves and their children. Ultimately, however, they could not promise that all mothers and children would share equally in that progress.

This study begins by examining the context from which health reform emerged in early twentieth-century Illinois as the peculiarities of gender, class, and regional distinctiveness shaped the contours of preventive health and hygiene campaigns. Chapter 2 looks more closely at Chicago health reformers' efforts to modernize the immigrant mother by transforming her Old World beliefs and practices into American ones and explores a range of responses from immigrant women themselves. A shift in focus to the downstate region of Illinois in chapter 3 highlights the subtext of modernization underlying rural health reform campaigns seeking to enlist the support of affluent farm women. Chapter 4 investigates the links between the use of modern media and the message of health reform in the displays, exhibits, mechanical models, and films that extended preventive health and hygiene education into communities throughout the state. Chapter 5 analyzes the severe political tensions that erupted in the early 1920s over federal sponsorship for maternal and child health programs and the significant shift in the emphasis of health reform represented by this conflict. A brief epilogue considers the legacy the early twentieth-century health reform movement in Illinois left in its wake.

1

Health and Modernity:
Preventive Health Reform in
Progressive Era Illinois

In July 1909 volunteers for the Chicago Department of Public Health walked door-to-door through that city's poorest tenement districts, inquiring of mothers at every household whether they had an ailing child at home. All that month representatives of local private philanthropies including the United Charities, the Elizabeth McCormick Memorial Fund, and the Visiting Nurse Association canvassed the city's hot and steamy streets and winding back alleys, urging mothers to bring their sick children to neighborhood infant welfare stations before it was too late to save the little ones. At the same time, an army of volunteers raised funds to support the operation of free clinics where babies could be weighed and measured to ensure they were developing properly. Ongoing educational programs in several different languages demonstrated the precepts of infant hygiene to poor and working-class mothers throughout the city.

Every year in Chicago, thousands of young children perished from severe dehydration resulting from "summer complaint," the common name given to a variety of children's diarrheal diseases which ravaged the city during the hottest months of the year. A 1909 study conducted by the University of Chicago Settlement revealed that of 1,330 patients brought to health clinics that summer, 542 (41%) presented symptoms of infection in the intestinal tract. In July of that year health care workers reported being "overwhelmed" by the number of young cases brought to their attention. "For many years in Chicago no large organized effort for the control of diarrhea had been undertaken," recalled Dr. Caroline Hedger, a recent graduate of Chicago's Rush Medical College who authored the study. "We calmly accepted the annual harvest of death as if it were inevitable as the weather, as if indeed a part of the weather." Although activities promoting public health had been underway for decades in Chicago, this kind of direct, intensive, and

Table 1.1
Deaths of Children as a Percentage of All Deaths in
Illinois, 1860–1880

Census Year	Under 1 Year	Under 5 Years
1860	22.8	51.4
1870	27.3	50.3
1880	24.0	43.0

Source: Rawlings, The Rise and Fall of Disease in Illinois (1927), pp.
97–99, 378.

proactive approach to combatting high rates of childhood death was new.
With the founding of the Infant Welfare Society of Chicago in 1911, such a
progressive strategy became a permanent feature of the city's social welfare
efforts. Just one year later, the society recorded caring for a total of 3,423
children at seven well-baby clinics in a number of wards; within ten years, it
had established twenty centers where volunteers examined more than 11,000
children each year.[1] An ambitious, widespread campaign to save Chicago's
youngest residents was now in full swing.

Historically, children had paid the highest price for poor public health
conditions in Chicago, as they had throughout the remainder of Illinois. In
the mid-1800s, children under five years of age had represented fully half of
all deaths occurring annually in the state (table 1.1). Each year between 1843
and 1872, children under five accounted for over 50 percent of all deaths
that occurred in Chicago; in 1871, this proportion topped 70 percent. The
proportion of early childhood deaths in Chicago (63%) was higher than the
proportion found in New York (49%) or New Orleans (32%); it was also considerably higher than the national figure, which stood at 41 percent.[2]

Every year, the incidence of gastrointestinal illness and death among
young children rose precipitously during the hot summer months. In the
1870s, for example, death rates for Chicago children under five years old
were four times higher in July than in the winter months. While popular
domestic manuals offered mothers all manner of advice on how best to alle-
viate their children's suffering, the etiology of gastrointestinal diseases in infants and young children remained only very poorly understood. Physicians
and parents alike associated the sudden, unexplained onset of diarrhea, or
"cholera infantum," with teething in infants, and mothers anxiously attended their babies throughout the dentition process. A variety of hypotheses

purporting to explain this alarming seasonal phenomenon circulated throughout the medical community. In 1871, for example, a physician addressing the Illinois State Medical Society believed he had identified the cause of summer diarrhea as a paralysis of the central nervous system due to excessively hot weather. The following year, the Chicago Board of Health listed "teething" as one of the leading causes of childhood death in that city.[3]

By the time Illinois entered the twentieth century, the persistence of high rates of childhood disease and death despite improvements in the overall death rate alarmed many reformers. Public health officials in Chicago consistently recorded higher infant mortality rates than did their colleagues in other northern industrial cities, a sorry state of affairs that did not sit well with progressive city boosters eager to promote the modern advantages of their city. In 1916, for example, Chicago's death rate for children under two years of age was 141.4 per 1,000 live births, as compared with 129.3 recorded for Detroit, 88.3 for Philadelphia, 58.1 for New York, and 49.4 for Boston. More than one-third of all deaths of children under two were attributed to diarrheal diseases.[4] "Enteritis under 2" remained as one of the top ten causes of death reported by the Illinois State Board of Health each year from 1902 to 1913, and dramatic increases in childhood diarrheal diseases continued to be identified during the hot summer months. Between 1912 and 1918, the Chicago Department of Health reported that, of the 58,575 infant deaths that occurred in the city, more than 36 percent had succumbed due to diarrheal diseases.[5]

Progressive reformers expressed dismay that the health hazards that had plagued Chicago's children since its days as a frontier town persisted into the new century. In the mid-1800s, Chicago's sanitarian health reformers had been convinced that "miasmas" or foul odors emanating from the polluted Chicago River represented a major source of ill health and untimely death among the city's population. Public health officials therefore devised an amazingly ambitious plan to carry waste out of the city by reversing the direction of the Chicago River's flow, an engineering venture that worked only imperfectly at best. Periodic heavy rains raised the river and caused it to resume its natural course, emptying tons of sewage and industrial waste into Lake Michigan, the main source of the city's drinking water. Continuing public pressure to clean up the odious river forced the Illinois General Assembly in Springfield to create an entirely new agency, the Chicago Sanitary District, in 1889. Eleven years later, the completion of a massive drainage canal diverted the city's sewage away from Lake Michigan, effecting a noticeable improvement in sanitary conditions. A series of smaller canals virtually eliminated malaria in the entire northern third of the state; outbreaks of cholera and typhoid fever also declined appreciably in this area.[6]

As promising as such developments were, however, serious public health problems persisted among sizable segments of the city's population. Black Chicagoans, for example, died of tuberculosis at a rate that was six times that of whites, while pneumonia and venereal diseases remained endemic to many neighborhoods, both black and white. Mothers of young children still anticipated the hot summer months with dread. Death rates from such maladies seemed stubbornly intractable despite the significant advancements in Chicago's public health environment realized through large-scale sanitation measures.

Meanwhile, a parallel movement of well-organized and energetic women had organized to combat the "harvest of death" that continued to plague Chicago's youngest residents. Drawing upon a maternalist cultural assumption that granted all women a special prerogative in matters concerning mothers and children, women had entered new professional fields such as public health, home economics, and social work and were now initiating spirited campaigns to improve children's physical well-being in their city. They were joined in their efforts by thousands of other women who, although not professionally trained, also used the ideology of maternalism as a springboard for their participation in public life. Women's club members, for example, had taken their obligations in safeguarding the public's health very seriously since the nineteenth century.

While Chicago's medical schools did not teach pediatrics as a specialty until the 1880s, almost twenty years earlier the elite Chicago Woman's Club had provided crucial financial and social support for the opening of a special hospital for poor women and children. Within five years of its founding in 1865 by Mary H. Thompson — the first female graduate to receive a degree from the Chicago Medical College — the Hospital for Women and Children became the city's premier training site for women medical students. Connections between the Chicago Woman's Club and local female physicians remained close ("we had always been partial to women in medicine," the club's longtime president, Sara L. Hart, recalled in her memoirs), and a number of medical doctors could be found listed among the club's membership rolls. Physicians Julia Holmes Smith and Sarah Hackett Stevenson each served terms as president of the Chicago Woman's Club; its members were also instrumental in the appointment of a woman, Dr. Dales Howe, to look after female inmates of the Cook County Insane Asylum. In 1915, the club underwrote internist Caroline Hedger's six-month tour of duty caring for young typhoid fever victims in war-torn Belgium.

Elite Chicago women donated an average of $69,000 to local facilities each year between 1900 and 1909, a sum that exceeded the amount they gave to cultural or educational projects.[7] Significantly, Chicago women's philanthropic activities were not limited solely to aiding established medical institutions in the city, for many of their projects actually represented innovative new measures in the delivery of health care. In June 1880, for example, Chicago Woman's Club members organized the Woman's Physiological Institute of Chicago for the purpose of "giving lectures on babies and hygiene for mothers and infants"; in 1903 this organization became the Children's Hospital Society, an active sponsor of health reform activities in the city. In 1889, twelve "women of social prominence" founded the Visiting Nurse Association of Chicago, modeling their organization after the district nursing system in London. The Visiting Nurse Association soon became one of the most important public health agencies in the city. Chicago women assumed a highly visible role in civic affairs when the Municipal Order League, under the leadership of Ada Celeste Sweet, launched a massive crusade to clean up the city in time for the World's Columbian Exposition in 1893.[8] Ellen Henrotin, president of the Chicago Woman's Club from 1902 to 1903, personally "devised, financed and superintended" a special traveling exhibit on infant hygiene during the spring of 1909. One of Chicago's wealthiest residents, Harriet Hammond McCormick, established the Elizabeth McCormick Memorial Fund in 1908 to honor her daughter who had died of pneumonia at the age of twelve. The fund supported "experimental and pioneer work" in children's health care, including visiting nurse services, "fresh air schools," and well-baby clinics throughout the city.[9] After 1911, the women's auxiliary of the Infant Welfare Society of Chicago provided vital publicity and fund-raising support for the organization's activities. The society also received valuable assistance from the Woman's City Club of Chicago; the two organizations cooperated, for example, in maintaining a children's health center in the twenty-second ward on the city's north side.[10]

In the first decades of the twentieth century medical researchers and maternalist reformers became increasingly aware of the specific causal relationships between poor maternal health and early infant death. As a result, the focus of "baby-saving" broadened to include the goal of "mother-saving" as well. Infants whose mothers died in childbirth, studies conducted by the United States Children's Bureau showed, were three to five times more likely to succumb than those whose mothers survived. Neonatal mortality (deaths of infants under thirty days old) from such factors as prematurity and low birth weight — causes rooted in the prenatal period — actually appeared to be on the increase. Nationally, complications due to childbirth represented one of the most frequent causes of death among all adult women in this era; rates of maternal death, in fact, remained frustratingly stable from 1915 to 1935.[11]

This dismal situation was reflected in Illinois, where childbirth-related causes followed only tuberculosis as the most frequent cause of death for adult women. In the nineteenth century, the considerable hazards of pregnancy and childbearing confronted by all women had been compounded by the deadly fevers female settlers had encountered on the midwestern prairies. In 1836, homesteader Eliza M. Farnham traveled from New York to start a new life with her sister in Tazewell County, Illinois. Farnham arrived only to find herself in the midst of a virulent fever epidemic. A published memoir, *Life in Prairie Land*, recounts the sad plight of her sister's nearest neighbors, a household in which a young woman and her stillborn infant became two of the epidemic's most unfortunate victims. "The babe that had been so long and joyfully expected," Farnham related, "was thrown heedlessly aside, and all attention concentrated on the sinking mother — but vainly. She survived only till the third day."[12]

But conditions for childbearing women were equally alarming in the growing city of Chicago. Between 1856 and 1896, Chicago Board of Health officials identified infection immediately following childbirth as the cause of death for 13 percent of all women who died between the ages of twenty and fifty. Major improvements had not been realized even well into the twentieth century. As late as 1914, of the 4,681 women of childbearing age who died in Chicago, tuberculosis claimed the lives of 1,078 (23%) while puerperal causes claimed the second largest number, 392 (8%).[13]

The virtual absence of prenatal medical services at this time meant that serious medical conditions such as an ectopic pregnancy (implantation of the fertilized egg in a fallopian tube rather than the uterus) or eclampsia (a drastic increase in blood pressure) usually went undetected until they became life-threatening. Chicago Department of Health mortality records, for example, listed complications of the prenatal period such as "ectopic pregnancies," "albuminuria and convulsions," and "sudden death in pregnancy" among the identifiable causes of maternal death in the city; Chicago records also reveal that a significant number of adult female deaths in this period were due to illegal abortions. But by far the greatest number of maternal deaths resulted from infections contracted during or shortly after childbirth. Of the 352 maternal deaths recorded in Chicago during 1912, for example, septicemia (infection) was identified as the primary cause in 124 cases (35%), a proportion that exceeded national averages at this time. The Chicago Community Trust estimated that each year from 1912 to 1920 five to six mothers died for every 1,000 live births, a deplorable state of affairs that seemed to belie civic boosters' claims about the extent of progress that had been achieved in their city since its frontier days.[14] In response, Chicago maternalists organized to address the health needs of parturient women in their city. While just four prenatal clinics had been established prior to 1900 (located at the Mary H. Thompson Hospital, Chicago Lying-In Hospital, Central Free Dispensary, and Chicago Polyclinic), during the period from 1910 to 1920 alone another nineteen such clinics opened in various locations throughout the city.[15]

Although individuals from all socioeconomic classes experienced the untimely deaths of family members in the early twentieth century, some of the highest maternal and childhood mortality rates in Chicago were recorded in districts heavily populated by poor and working-class immigrants. A 1910 survey conducted in the nineteenth ward, a predominantly Russian and Italian district, found death rates of children under one year of age ranging from 183 to over 300 per 1,000 live births.[16] Nowhere in the city were the rates of infant death higher than in Packingtown, an area of approximately three square miles inhabited by 45,000 people, mostly industrial meatpacking workers and their families. Packingtown's unhealthfulness was legendary. A 1902 survey found that the overall death rate in this district was 55 percent higher than the average for the city as a whole. Tuberculosis in the poorly constructed, overcrowded tenements constituted an ever-present menace; sanitary facilities for the families living in many of these structures remained crude. In 1906 Caroline Hedger described a house call she had made in Packingtown, a visit to a dark and airless basement apartment in order to attend a boy afflicted with tuberculosis of the spine. "Children in such surroundings," Hedger remarked with her characteristic candor, "have just about as much chance for life and stamina as a potato sprout in a cellar." Sadly, the young patient in this account did not survive.[17]

Perhaps the most deadly threat to the public's health in Packingtown, however, came from "Bubbly Creek," a stagnant branch of the Chicago River into which flowed refuse from no less than nineteen different meatpacking plants, turning the creek into one large open sewer. Mary McDowell, head resident of the University of Chicago Settlement, which had been established in the district in 1894, bristled with frustration over the callousness of local officials toward this ever-present threat to the public's health:

We were shocked, during one discussion at City Hall, to hear a lawyer of education and refinement say in his argument: "Gentlemen, you know in all large cities there must be a place segregated for unpleasant things, and of course the people living there are not sensitive." The room was filled with those of us who lived in just such a district segregated for unpleasant things.[18]

Settlement workers and public health officials, of course, were not the only area residents keenly aware of Packingtown's abysmal environment. Evidence from the neighborhood's inhabitants themselves, a community of predominantly Polish, Lithuanian, and Bohemian immigrants, attests to their own "sensitivity" to the overcrowding, ever-present dirt, and oppressive odors they experienced on a daily basis. One woman recalled the shock of encountering for the first time the dismal surroundings of her new home, a tenement dwelling constructed near Bubbly Creek in the shadow of the Wilson and Company meatpacking plant. "That was stockyards, you know, smelling," she remembered many years later, "and then I thought to myself, that priest said the truth, this is hell."[19] Under such deplorable circumstances, then, mothers and babies fought an uphill battle for survival. Mary McDowell estimated that Packingtown's immigrant communities lost nearly one out of every three children before they reached their second birthday; the infant mortality rate in Packingtown stood at seven and one-half times that for affluent Hyde Park.[20]

In 1908, Caroline Hedger launched an investigation into the ongoing public health hazards of Packingtown, where "whirling, choking clouds of dust swept off the streets and penetrated not only yards but houses." She found 127 cases of diarrheal disease within an area measuring one-fourth of a square mile, all of them children under the age of five. The afflicted children appeared to be suffering from severe dehydration, a potentially deadly condition that Hedger felt to be exacerbated by the behavior of immigrant mothers themselves, as "the Slavic people seem to have a national prejudice against giving a baby water to drink." Hedger expressed amazement that some very careful mothers were indeed managing to rear apparently healthy children — almost miraculously — "against the odds of dirt, crowding, and lack of bathing facilities" that typified Packingtown's tenement environment. A great many others, however, appeared to be losing the battle. "They love their babies," Hedger concluded sympathetically, "but with no money for doctors, milk so expensive they cannot buy it, the ever-present dirt and overhanging smoke of the yards, what can they do?"[21] Tragically, but perhaps not surprisingly, Packingtown ranked first among all of the city's wards in female death rates from causes connected with childbirth. In the absence of infection-fighting drugs, of course, the specter of severe complications from

puerperal septicemia haunted all childbearing women in this period, regardless of their social class, place of residence, or whether they gave birth in a
hospital or their own home. But, under the infamously unsanitary conditions
of Chicago's poorest tenement districts, infection posed a grave hazard for
immigrant mothers.[22]

Recent discoveries in bacteriology meant that a number of illnesses
could now be linked directly to water and food supplies. A series of investigations during the period from 1890 to 1910 had revealed the role played by
vectors, or intermediaries, in the etiology of disease. The spread of contagious illness through milk, for example, had received increased attention
from medical researchers and public health authorities since this alarming
possibility had first been proposed at London's International Medical Congress in 1881.[23] The identification of contaminated milk as a major cause
of childhood illness and death added an important new dimension to the
campaign against diarrheal diseases in Chicago.

Although municipal ordinances had prohibited the sale of "swill" and
adulterated milk since the 1870s, health officials warned that city milk supplies continued to be infected by bacteria at unsanitary dairies operating in
outlying rural areas. They also charged that milk was being contaminated
after arriving in the city by unscrupulous distributors who adulterated the
product with impure water or ice; a small percentage of samples in the city's
testing program had been discovered to contain formaldehyde, which some
distributors had been adding to the milk as a preservative. In 1903, as an
outgrowth of the extensive child welfare activities carried out by the Chicago
Woman's Club, a special Milk Commission began overseeing the distribution of pasteurized milk at low cost to needy families throughout the city.
Settlement houses, including Hull House, Chicago Commons, and Northwestern University, served as the principal distribution centers for the Milk
Commission, dispensing thousands of the eight-ounce bottles during the hot
summer months. In 1908, Chicago became the first municipality in the
world to mandate the pasteurization of its milk supply; by 1910, a complex set
of ordinances had been put into place to regulate milk in that city. Chicago's
nefarious water supply underwent chemical treatment for the first time in
1913.[24]

The growing sophistication with which Illinois health reformers understood the spread of contagious diseases in the early twentieth century had
important ramifications for small towns and rural villages outside of Chicago
as well. Lacking both a public health infrastructure and an organized maternalist movement to advocate for reform, rural areas lagged distinctly behind

Chicago in realizing improvements. Throughout the nineteenth century the state's southernmost portion had been especially notorious for its unhealthfulness. Steamy hot summers, marshy terrain, and frequent flooding from the Mississippi and Illinois rivers rendered maladies such as yellow fever, cholera, and dysentery endemic to the region.

Early settlers pushing westward from New England and the mid-Atlantic states generally avoided what came to be known ignominiously as "Egypt," an allusion to the area's periodic flooding. After touring southern Illinois in 1842, British novelist Charles Dickens related his negative impressions of the river town of Cairo in no uncertain terms:

> A dismal swamp, on which the half-built houses rot away; cleared here and there for the space of a few yards; and teeming, then, with rank, unwholesome vegetation, in whose baleful shade the wretched wanderers who are tempted hither droop, and die, and lay their bones; the hateful Mississippi circling and eddying before it, and turning off upon its southern course, a slimy monster hideous to behold; a hotbed of disease, an ugly sepulchre, a grave uncheered by any gleam of promise: a place without one single quality, in earth or air or water, to commend it: such is this dismal Cairo.[25]

Dickens, in fact, had been so stricken by the harrowing health conditions he had encountered on his travels in southern Illinois that he later worked them into the plot of his novel *Martin Chuzzlewit*. His impressions can be corroborated by evidence from medical officers' journals at the United States Marine Hospital Service Relief Station in Cairo that also chronicle continuous cycles of dysentery, typhoid fever, diphtheria, meningitis, malaria, and influenza along with shootings, stabbings, and bouts with venereal disease they routinely treated among the local population. "Weather worse than yesterday," one officer reported on a hot August day in 1882, "almost everyone in town is sick." Four years later, the officer noted that "there is a great deal of smallpox, scarlet fever and diphtheria on the other side of the river between here and Memphis, Tennessee."[26]

Even the Illinois Central Railroad found its efforts to colonize the southern region thwarted when upstate newspaper editors warned farmers not to be tempted by the railroad's offers of cheap land. During the middle decades of the nineteenth century, enterprising easterners hoping to establish commercial crop farms on the rich midwestern prairies continued to avoid the extreme southern portion of Illinois, leaving the area to be settled instead by migrating southerners who by and large resisted the transition to capitalist farming. "But very few from the Northern and Eastern states," reported the *Cairo Weekly Times* in 1856, "could be induced to explore [southern Illinois] and judge from personal inspection of the truth or falsity of the current statements reflecting it."[27]

As agricultural development in the northernmost portion of the state outpaced that in the south, a clear divergence between northern and southern Illinois became apparent. By 1849, for example, 72 percent of all Illinois farms were located in the north; further, northern farms accounted for 83 percent of the total dollar value of land and machinery in the state. Technological innovations such as the building of the Illinois and Michigan Canal and the proliferation of railroads greatly stimulated agricultural development, but commercial farming developed unevenly throughout the state. By 1870, the average farm enterprise in southern Illinois produced one-third less and was only half as valuable as its northern counterpart. Former slaves also began to migrate northward into Illinois, establishing permanent communities in three counties at the extreme southern end of the state: Pulaski, Massac, and Alexander. By 1900, African Americans constituted 40 percent of the population of Pulaski County, situated along the state's border with Kentucky, making it the largest rural black community in the north. Economic, social, and cultural disparities between the extreme ends of the state were now well established. "Yankee" farmers in northern Illinois wrote to the influential midwestern journal *The Prairie Farmer* complaining of the "backwardness" of southern counties.[28] To many northerners, the region's continued public health problems in the wake of identifiable progress in the north only provided further evidence for their prejudices.

Residents of southern Illinois counties grappled with frequent outbreaks of infectious disease well into the twentieth century. Typhoid fever, the "filth disease," remained a well-known if unwelcome visitor to this region, and as late as 1914 numerous cases of malaria and smallpox were still being recorded at the Marine Hospital Service Relief Station in Cairo. To their surprise, Illinois health reformers found tuberculosis—a disease many associated with overcrowded urban slum conditions characteristic of Chicago's most blighted tenement districts—to be endemic in the open countryside as well. In 1915, the Illinois State Board of Health began issuing special cards to local and district health officers in an attempt to more accurately pinpoint the sources and modes of infectious disease in rural areas. During an epidemic, local public health officers used the cards to record data such as the origins

of the community's milk and water supplies and the names of schools attended by all infected children. The information reported could then be
compiled to map the epidemic's trajectory. That year the central region of
Illinois was hit by over two hundred cases of typhoid fever, the source of
which health officials eventually traced to polluted wells at the Old Salem
Chautauqua held in August.[29]

In July of 1916 the town of Tuscola (with a population of approximately
2,400) experienced an outbreak of typhoid fever that spread quickly throughout the surrounding areas of Douglas County, reaching a total of 110 cases
before it had subsided. Public health officials eventually traced the source
of the epidemic to a single well with defective walls; water from this well
had been utilized in many private homes, as well as by the local druggist,
confectioner, and the owner of the town hotel. The leaking well was located
near the privy vault of a livery stable, leading the public health officials who
investigated the outbreak to presume that the disease originated with a trav-
eler passing through the town. The Tuscola epidemic proved instructive to
Illinois health reformers in that it demonstrated unequivocally the dangers
posed by contaminated water supplies in the country. "Even the graduate in
sanitary science or the man loaded to the guards with theoretical training,"
the State Board of Health asserted, "will find that there is much for him to
observe and much for him to learn" from such rural episodes.[30] Armed with
a new understanding of the etiology of contagious disease, Illinois health
reformers were hopeful that the egregiously poor public health conditions
that had plagued the downstate region since Dickens's day could at last be
corrected.

But while dramatic, periodic visitations of disease served as an important source of scientific enlightenment in the early twentieth century, it was
actually the deplorable state of wells and household cisterns found on many
farms that led health reformers to brand contaminated water supplies as the
"great menace of the rural community" (figure 1.1). "The general sanitary
conditions are often unspeakable," declared Dr. Thomas D. Wood, chairman of the National Council of Education's Committee on Health Problems which, in 1917, undertook a major survey of rural health conditions in
cooperation with the American Medical Association. "The disposal of waste
matter dangerous to health is frequently ignored. The fly as an active carrier
of germs is also frequently ignored. And the same can be said of drainage,
with the result that there are many damp cellars and musty houses. Country
water is often contaminated. The barnyard and the primitive cesspool for
household purposes are too frequently placed without reference to the well,

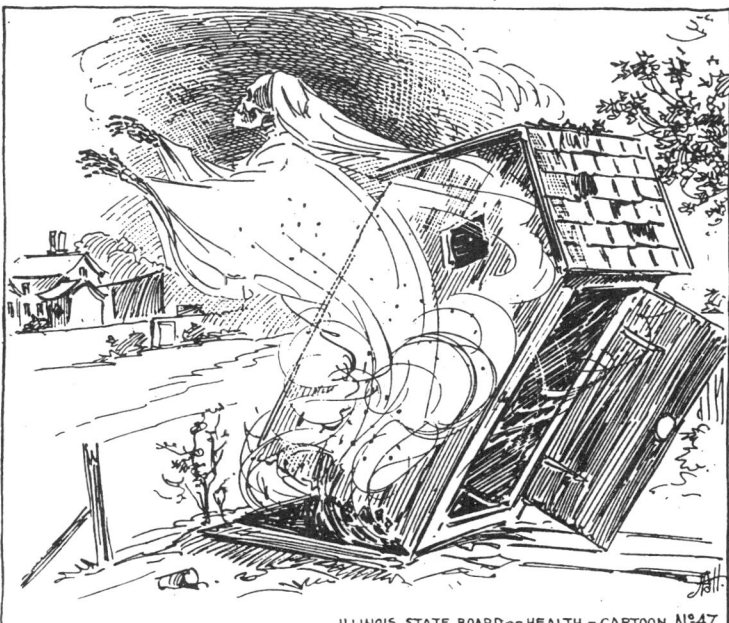

Figure 1.1. Illinois State Department of Public Health cartoon dramatically illustrating the dangers posed by unsanitary water supplies in rural areas. *Illinois Health News*, December 1916.

spring, or brook that supplies the drinking water." Census data show that as late as 1920 only 11 percent of Illinois farm families had plumbing installed in their homes.[31]

Investigations into rural water supplies carried out by the Illinois State Water Survey discovered numerous cases in which farm wells that provided household water supplies were located just a few yards from outdoor privies, cesspools, and stables. Shallow wells posed particular health dangers in that the water source could easily become contaminated from seepage on the surface, particularly after a bout of heavy rain. But digging new wells was an expensive enterprise and therefore farmers preferred to reuse contaminated wells, simply digging an additional few feet to the source of groundwater.[32] In addition, many farm families continued to rely on cisterns, commonly located at the top of the farmhouse in order to collect rainwater, as their primary source of drinking water. In 1915, a University of Illinois study found that 68 percent of all the farm homes surveyed used cisterns for their water supply. Although rural dwellers generally preferred to drink cistern water because it tasted "sweeter" than the mineral-rich water obtained from wells, cisterns that were not kept meticulously clean could eventually build up high levels of disease-causing bacteria. Since contaminated water often *looked* perfectly clear and had no odor, farm families had no way of recognizing danger. Children's "summer complaint" and a variety of other gastrointestinal illnesses often became the unfortunate result.[33]

Most health reformers in Illinois believed that the poor public health environments they documented in the country posed particular problems for mothers and children. The conditions under which a great many farm women bore children in their own homes remained far from sanitary, and the ongoing hazard of "childbed fever" constituted nearly as severe a threat to parturient women in the country as it did in the city. Because the initial discoveries revealing that puerperal septicemia could be transmitted from patient to patient by medical practitioners had been made in urban hospitals, nineteenth-century sanitarians had not immediately associated this danger with rural childbearing practices, which by tradition involved deliveries at home with few (or no) outside attendants. Twentieth-century investigators of rural health conditions began to discover, however, that the problem of infection following childbirth may have been greater in the country than was generally realized. Because few states mandated the official reporting of puerperal sepsis as a specific cause of death, rural localities frequently recorded childbearing women as dying of other causes including septic pneumonia, "cryptogenic" (of unknown causes) infection, or even tuberculosis.[34]

Health reformers believed that the young were particularly at risk as well, as bacteriological infection from contaminated water and milk supplies in rural areas could be especially dangerous for infants and small children. Although individuals eventually built up immunities to local bacteria, those newly exposed could contract serious illnesses. Babies who had not yet acquired sufficient immunities were extremely susceptible to water- and milk-borne diseases, as were young children whose immune systems had become compromised through an illness, even a relatively minor one. While a young baby's diet normally did not include ingesting large quantities of water, even very small amounts of contaminated water may have caused severe illness in babies who were especially small or weak. Water was, of course, also used in the preparation of many foods fed to young children, and bacteria could thus be transferred from contaminated water to media that were even more conducive to their growth.[35]

The milk consumed by rural dwellers in Illinois remained virtually unregulated in the early twentieth century. Despite Chicago's early lead in requiring pasteurization of the milk supply, regulating the dairy industry proved to be a political minefield in Illinois; by 1920 only nineteen milk testing associations operated outside of Chicago. A model milk supply ordinance developed jointly by the State Department of Public Health and the Department of Agriculture at the University of Illinois was not put forward until 1922; local approval of the ordinance in sixty Illinois municipalities took an additional five years.[36]

Despite these glaring problems, the paucity of downstate public health services meant that local residents often had to take health reform into their own hands. White County is located at the southeastern corner of the state, separated from Indiana by the Wabash River. In 1915 a small group of "progressive and wide-awake" White County citizens, alarmed by what appeared to be an abnormally high rate of tuberculosis among the predominantly white and overwhelmingly rural population of approximately 23,000, wrote to the Illinois State Board of Health requesting a health survey in their county. Many school children, these concerned citizens claimed, appeared "pale and anemic" and had a strong family history of tuberculosis. In addition, diseases such as smallpox, malaria, and measles visited White County with disturbing regularity. The survey was undertaken by Dr. I. A. Foster, a medical inspector for the Illinois State Board of Health, and Harriet Fulmer, a former superintendent of the Visiting Nurse Association of Chicago who now represented the Illinois State Association for the Prevention of Tuberculosis. Fulmer was instrumental in establishing an outdoor camp for tuberculosis sufferers in Glencoe, Illinois.[37]

Upon concluding their investigation, Foster and Fulmer reported finding

a strange sort of overall malaise or lethargy that seemed to afflict a high proportion of White County's residents. They estimated that fully 25 percent of
schoolchildren were "anemic and undernourished," a condition that also
appeared to be a general characteristic of the community at large. "Many
young people," the surveyors observed, "were found to be 'just dragging
around' as they term it." While Foster and Fulmer did not speculate on the
etiology of this chronic malady, they did express alarm at the extremely unsanitary conditions they had found in a great many White County homes.
Houses tended to be very small in proportion to the number of residents
dwelling in them, a finding that seemed more characteristic of urban tenement districts than of this overwhelmingly rural area. The majority of county
residents still used outdoor privies, and the high number of unsanitary ones,
related the investigators, was "well-nigh unbelievable." Foster and Fulmer
deemed only four of the 119 privies they inspected to be "fairly decent"; forty-
two were reportedly "so filthy and unsanitary as to be an absolute menace to
the neighborhood." Most of the houses they inspected were equipped with
rooftop cisterns; the investigators were concerned but not surprised to find
that one farming community encompassing an area of less than two and one-
half square miles contained no fewer than seventeen cases of typhoid fever.[38]

Although many of the problems Foster and Fulmer uncovered were the
result of unfortunate local environmental conditions, including a dearth of
fresh water supplies and inadequately drained soils, they nevertheless placed
a significant portion of the blame on the behavior of White County residents
themselves. Foster and Fulmer pointed to the "backwardness" of southern
Illinoisans in general, concluding that many of the area's deplorable public
health problems ensued from a general "disregard of all duty toward their
neighbors" that kept locals from taking the most basic sanitary precautions
such as boiling their drinking water. They ascribed nutritional deficiencies
to residents' customary avoidance of fresh vegetables rather than a lack of
availability; further, these urban-based investigators asserted there existed
a "positive dislike for sunshine and fresh air" among White County inhabitants. They even went so far as to suggest that a high degree of "feeble-
mindedness and physical deterioration" in area residents had been the unfortunate result of generations of "consanguineous marriage."

Foster and Fulmer were especially dismayed at the number of White
County residents who apparently relied heavily on patent medicines and attempted dangerous self-help cures in order to relieve their chronic ailments.
"Calomel and quinine are taken without prescription," they reported, "and
patent medicines are found to an alarming extent in every farmhouse

throughout the county." One destitute family's bill for medicines, which had been paid by the county supervisors, included Piso's Consumption Cure, Wine of Cardui, and Mrs. Winslow's Soothing Syrup (an opium derivative). Perceptively, Foster and Fulmer also noted that White County was a "dry" district, and the popularity of patent medicines among its residents led these investigators to question "whether the prohibition law carries with it all that one might expect"; a number of restaurants reportedly sold intoxicating soft drinks as well.

Interestingly, it was young women in White County who apparently imbibed patent medicines containing alcohol most frequently. One patient, reportedly in the terminal stage of tuberculosis, confessed that she drank Wine of Cardui "on account of its stimulant effect." Another woman told the investigators that, although she had seen a number of doctors for her ailments, "they did not know what they were talking about," and she continued to use Piso's Consumption Cure because it "at least made her comfortable." (Unfortunately, they did not hazard an opinion in their published report as to why it was young women among White County residents who seemed to be especially reliant on alcoholic remedies.) While harsh in their condemnation of "backward" behavior among these southern Illinoisans, Foster and Fulmer also castigated public health officials for their "lack of personal courage" and their failure to assume responsibility for chronic health problems in the county. They concluded their report with an urgent call for the installation of "a salaried health officer to enforce health laws without fear or favor."[39]

Some of the most serious health hazards in rural Illinois existed within the various coal mining communities located throughout the state. Bituminous coal mining had been carried out in Illinois since the nineteenth century. A mining boom from 1900 to 1910 saw the opening of many new fields in quick succession, and for the next ten years Illinois stood as the nation's second leading coal-producing state, following Pennsylvania. These new fields, located predominantly in southern counties, were worked primarily by immigrant miners, especially Italians, Lithuanians, and Russians. Williamson County, for example, saw its mining population grow from 1,440 in 1910 to 7,760 in 1920, nearly half of whom were foreign-born. Although the majority of the immigrants had been farm laborers in Europe, many preferred to work in the mines because they lacked the necessary capital to establish their own farms in the United States; in addition, coal mining paid higher wages than did hired farm labor in Illinois.[40]

In 1919 Grace Abbott, a former resident of Hull House now serving as

the Executive Secretary of the Illinois Immigrants Commission, surveyed
coal mining communities in Williamson, Franklin, Bureau, and Sangamon
counties. This study by the future head of the Children's Bureau revealed
considerable variation in the working and living conditions among the different mining sites. Although the survey was not designed to document public
health problems specifically, the sanitary conditions that Abbott uncovered
in the company towns proved to be appalling. At the Ziegler mine in Williamson County, for example, 3,500 people (including a large number of
Croats and Serbs) were housed in barracks owned and operated by the company. As many as thirty families lived under one roof, and in the seven years
that the camp had been in existence, Abbott discovered, *no* attempt had
been made by the company to either remove rubbish or clean outdoor toilet facilities.

Williamson and Franklin County miners and their families who did not
live in barracks lived in extremely small houses, the majority having four
rooms or less; 21 percent of these mining families housed boarders in these
overcrowded dwellings. Not one of the houses surveyed had an indoor water
supply, and Abbott found that residents were actually using water piped in
from the mines for bathing as well as drinking. As in the remainder of rural
Illinois, rooftop cisterns were common, but the miners' wives told Abbott
that during the area's frequent dry spells not enough water could be collected in them, a situation that forced these women to "get water wherever
they can" regardless of the safety of the source. "This carrying water from a
distance and having an insufficient supply," Abbott asserted, "adds to the
women's work, and it must also inevitably lower family standards of cleanliness." Sanitary conditions in the homes of mining families did in fact prove
to be grossly substandard.[41]

Illinois health reformers believed that continued social progress in their
state required concerted efforts to improve conditions in the countryside as
well as the city. Urban-based reformers expressed concern that a lack of sanitary precaution in rural areas could adversely affect city life as well. Many
Chicago dwellers already knew, for example, that traveling through the
downstate region for a few days might mean returning home with a case of
typhoid fever. But even more distressing was the prospect of deadly commu-
nicable diseases being imported wholesale into the city along with unregulated dairy milk and unwashed produce from the country. "The farmer's
illness, suffering, bills, and possible grief can thus be made our illness, suffering, bills, and possible grief," cautioned the social reform magazine *Outlook*
in 1917. The very survival of American cities depended on a constant — and

safe — supply of food brought in from the surrounding countryside; thus, many public health advocates warned that rural conditions should be of the utmost concern to country and city dwellers alike. The interdependence of town and country life in the modern age rendered rural public health reform an important issue in Progressive Era Illinois.[42]

But the unifying potential of wide-ranging health reform efforts in this period remained confined within distinct limits. Even as efforts to safeguard the health of mothers and children reached the height of their momentum in Chicago, the provision of health care services in that city remained sharply segregated by race. Although segregation had been officially outlawed in Chicago after 1880, a de facto color line was firmly in place.[43] Increasing migration from southern states, and to a lesser extent from the rural downstate region of Illinois as well, caused the city's African American population to expand rapidly in this period. During the decade from 1910 to 1920, for example, the black population of Chicago increased by 148.5 percent while the city's white population, by contrast, grew by just 21 percent. During one eighteen-month period in 1917–1918, more than 50,000 African Americans migrated to Chicago to work in the city's war industries. The sharp upswing in black migration to the city during these years placed additional strains on the already precarious public health conditions plaguing the poor and working-class neighborhoods of the city's overcrowded south side — districts to which the city's unofficial color line strictly confined newly arriving African Americans. On the national level, childhood and maternal mortality rates among African Americans in the early twentieth century exceeded those of whites by as much as 50 percent; recent demographic analyses have suggested that the single most important variable in predicting childhood mortality at this time was in fact race.[44]

Nevertheless, white reformers in Chicago remained overwhelmingly focused on poor public health conditions as a "foreign" problem being imported into their city by waves of recently arriving immigrants, especially those from southern and eastern Europe. Such a perspective allowed city public health officials and the supporters of Chicago's preventive health reform campaigns to ignore the equally pressing needs of native-born African Americans. Although the puerperal deaths recorded in Chicago during these years were not consistently categorized by race, a 1920 report by the Community Trust estimated that maternal mortality rates among black women in the city actually exceeded the alarmingly high national average, a tragic state of affairs that the trust attributed to the lack of high quality obstetrical care available to African Americans in Chicago. Interestingly, the report's authors concluded that, unlike foreign-born mothers who needed to be taught the value of health care services for their own and their children's well-being, native-born black mothers "require little education as to the value of good medical care at child-birth. Their very neglect has taught them their need." Many of Chicago's local health centers and neighborhood medical dispensaries either did not admit black patients at all or set aside a restricted number of hours for African Americans in order to keep them separated from their white clientele; some accepted black patients only if they had been brought into the facility by white staff members. Thus the problem of maternal and infant death among Chicago's black population persisted throughout the period described by historian Edward H. Beardsley as the "era of denial" in African American public health.[45]

It remained up to African Americans themselves, therefore, to fill the gaps left by white health reformers who reached out to European immigrants almost exclusively. Professionals and middle-class citizens from the city's black community developed a preventive health and hygiene movement that resembled but remained quite separate from the one supported by white Chicagoans. A significant portion of African American health reform activity in the early twentieth century revolved around Provident Hospital and Nurses' Training School, established in 1891 as the first black-controlled medical institution in the United States under the directorship of physician Daniel Hale Williams. The Nurses' Training School played a pivotal role in educating black nurses for public health work among Chicago's African American community in the early twentieth century.[46]

Like their white counterparts in health reform, black health care professionals and their middle-class allies in the African American community focused intensely on the education of mothers, especially poor mothers who had recently arrived in Chicago from the rural South, instructing them in the precepts of preventive health and hygiene as a key element in the bettering of health conditions in black neighborhoods. Practitioners at Provident, with support from local black women's organizations, supervised an infant feeding program for new mothers and operated a well-baby clinic within the hospital building, located at the corner of 29th and Dearborn streets.

Preventive health efforts in Chicago's African American community exhibited a strongly maternalist orientation as well. Building upon the solid groundwork established through the efforts of local women's clubs in a number of American cities, the African American public health movement quickly expanded via a national maternalist network comprised of mothers, midwives, nurses, teachers, home demonstration agents, and sorority members. Black women's work on behalf of public health reform in the early twentieth century became one important component within a more comprehensive program of self-help that included the founding of black colleges, orphanages, libraries, and recreational facilities.[47]

While white racism had engendered the need for African Americans to create separate institutions in the first place, it also served to shape the very ideological underpinnings of black public health and social welfare work in the early twentieth century. Black women activists, including those working in Chicago's preventive health campaigns, were forced to constantly defend African American home life against the charges of sexual and moral laxity that historically had been used to justify white liberal indifference toward blacks' social welfare and — in the face of widespread vigilante violence, especially in the South — toward their physical safety as well. "We are placed in the unfortunate position," asserted Chicago reformer Fannie Barrier Williams, "of being defenders of our name." (Williams's own vigorous efforts in the late nineteenth century had mobilized black community support for the establishment of the Nurses' Training School at Provident.)[48]

Given the pernicious influence of racist stereotypes, many middle-class health reformers in the African American community feared that persistently high rates of illness and death from causes regarded as largely preventable by this time could easily be dismissed by whites as yet another sign that black mothers were somehow failing in the proper conduct of their womanly duties. At the same time, the realities of racism in the early twentieth century meant that the economic and social gaps standing between black middle-class reformers and their poor and working-class clientele were considerably narrower than those between white health reform crusaders and immigrants from Europe. For many middle-class social welfare advocates, a demonstrable increase in clean homes, sanitary neighborhoods, and healthy children among the black population would serve as an indicator for measuring the success of their racial uplift efforts. House-to-house volunteers for the Urban League, for example, distributed preventive health instructions that in addition to promulgating personal cleanliness stressed sobriety and respectable behavior; the editors of the *Chicago Defender* admonished their readers that failure to follow modern methods of sanitation and hygiene could result in hostile commentary against "members of the race."[49] In racially segregated Chicago, black and white reformers developed essentially parallel preventive health and hygiene campaigns that shared a number of fundamental goals and strategies. As products of a racist society, however, these separate preventive health movements carried deeper social and political messages that prevented them from being identical.

Diverse in its manifestations, ambitious in its aims, and infused with the powerful ideological imperative of advancing social progress in the state, health reform in early twentieth-century Illinois extended its reach across both private and public spheres, from urban to rural communities, from the extreme northern to the extreme southern end of the state. By 1900, the obscurely understood and dreaded assortment of "fevers" once so central to life on the midwestern prairies had been brought largely under control in the state's northern regions, holding out a promise that realizing actual improvement in the general public health environment in Illinois was, in fact, an achievable goal.

Progress, however, had not been uniformly realized throughout the state. Serious health problems remained endemic to Chicago's poorest neighborhoods, including those occupied by recent immigrants from southern and eastern Europe and African Americans migrating from the rural South. To their dismay, the squalid conditions public health investigators found in many rural downstate communities seemed to have hardly changed since frontier days. Most galling of all to Illinois progressives was the stubborn persistence of high rates of maternal and infant mortality in their state, tragedies that reformers knew to be largely preventable in an age informed by the germ theory.

In response, a coalition of social welfare advocates, public health practitioners, elite philanthropists, and maternalist activists in urban and rural areas of the state united under a shared assumption that enlightened mothers need not stand by watching hopelessly as their little ones suffered and perished from sudden and mysterious ailments. Progressive health reformers brought to early twentieth-century campaigns an unwavering conviction that modern mothers, armed with the latest available information on preventive health and hygiene practices, could exert a degree of control over their own and their children's fate unimaginable to their grandmothers' generation.

2

Americanizing the Immigrant Mother

I n 1914, child health advocates working with the Elizabeth McCormick
Memorial Fund in Chicago set up a number of outdoor "baby tents" at
locations throughout the city to serve as makeshift clinics for tenement children taken ill during the oppressive heat and humidity of a midwestern summer. "Many mothers would walk back and forth past the tents several times
before they would yield to the desire to come in," reported one observer,

> Then, step by step, [the mothers] would let the baby be examined
> and cared for and perhaps placed in the tent. They would go away,
> only to reappear in a short time, walking hurriedly up the street.
> They could peer in at the door or come in, and when they found
> that the baby had not been spirited away, had not been operated
> upon, and nothing untoward had happened, they gradually ac-
> quired full confidence. This was the response of the mothers of the
> neighborhood.[1]

Health reformers in early twentieth-century Chicago envisioned themselves as mediators between the Old World and the New, for the movement
they created was as much about modernizing immigrant mothers' attitudes
and beliefs toward personal hygiene, household cleanliness, and the efficacy
of early intervention in keeping young children alive as it was about safeguarding the public's health. Middle-class, native-born activists in Chicago
directly linked their health reform efforts to the wider goal of acculturating
that city's immigrant communities, delineating through programs of preventive health and hygiene education a clear model of how their foreign-born
neighbors could come to live the "American way of life." Chicago reformers
believed their movement would serve as an important vehicle for instilling

in immigrant families what one health care organization described as a "desire for cleanliness of body, mind, and surroundings that they will imitate as American."[2] Under this model immigrant mothers, as the traditional health care practitioners within their own households, were to serve as the principal agents of change. But health reformers also determined that the very foreignness of the immigrant mother herself played a major part in the high rates of sickness and death consistently recorded in Chicago's immigrant wards. Thus they set out to replace foreign-born women's "superstitious" health care customs and "fatalistic" attitudes toward illness and death with a more modern — more appropriately American — faith in the efficacy of active intervention and the new credo of domestic hygiene. The "problem of the foreign mother" became a frequent topic of discussion at public health and social welfare conferences throughout the city.

Although a wide spectrum of Chicago organizations shared the view that the Americanization of immigrant mothers should represent a fundamental goal within health reform, groups remained somewhat divided regarding the sufficiency of such an approach for actually improving the state of immigrants' health. The maternalist activists associated with Hull House and the Chicago School of Civics and Philanthropy took a comprehensive view of health reform, pointing out that a wide range of physical and social variables affected maternal and infant mortality rates and calling for a multifaceted plan of attack on the tragic waste such rates represented. Soon after assuming leadership of the Children's Bureau, Hull House-trained Julia Lathrop launched a series of investigations that revealed an intricate interplay of factors affecting infant death rates in American industrial cities including low wages and unemployment, mothers' frequent childbearing, the length of time women recovered at home following childbirth, illiteracy, race, and ethnicity.[3] Despite the causal complexities that mounting evidence from the Children's Bureau seemed to suggest, however, local organizations in Chicago tended to stress ethnic and cultural differences as the key to stubbornly high mortality rates in their city. Dr. F. S. Churchill of the Infant Welfare Society of Chicago, for example, acknowledged the salience of poverty as a contributing factor in high rates of infant mortality, but deemed it less important than immigrant mothers' own ignorance of the germ theory in determining their children's fate.

For Churchill and other members of the philanthropic community, addressing the systemic causes of poverty in Chicago lay entirely outside their organizations' reach. Unlike preventive health and hygiene practices which could be taught to immigrant women, Churchill asserted, poverty itself was "impossible to eliminate. It will always be with us."[4] Such a perspective caused Grace Abbott, the director of the Immigrants Protective League who eventually would succeed Lathrop as chief of the Children's Bureau, to become discouraged at her Chicago colleagues' proclivity "to regard racial differences as the explanation of the infant mortality rate in a poor Polish or Italian district. It is always much easier to blame the immigrant than to face the economic and political causes that are really responsible." While they acknowledged factors such as the notoriously poor quality of tenement housing in Chicago and the unhealthful and hazardous working conditions in that city's burgeoning industries, locally based health reformers were much more likely to emphasize the "barriers of language, misunderstandings and prejudice" as the real culprits to be overcome in preventing the untimely deaths of immigrant mothers and children.[5]

But, if reformers envisioned the refashioning of Old World mothers into modern American ones, immigrant mothers themselves first needed to be convinced of the safety and efficacy of American-style health care practices before they would agree to exchange old wisdom for new. Deeply rooted cultural beliefs influenced the ways in which immigrant women themselves understood the causes of ill-health, how they evaluated the signs and symptoms of disease, the specific remedies they chose in order to ameliorate these symptoms, and to whom they would most likely turn for treatment when their family members did become ill. Evidence from medical anthropology suggests that customs and beliefs associated with pregnancy, birth, infant care, and food — the very things that Progressive Era health crusaders had targeted for transformation among Chicago's immigrant communities — carry very deep meanings in any culture and are especially resistant to change.[6] As native-born reformers and their foreign-born clientele met face-to-face at public health exhibits, neighborhood children's health clinics, and settlement house programs, the daily work of health reform unfolded as an intricate, ongoing process of negotiation. Through their continued questioning and doubt — as well as their active participation and willingness to exchange old customs for new — immigrant mothers also helped to shape health reform campaigns in significant ways.[7]

Immigrant women were free to accept or reject the health care advice reformers gave them. Although health care workers frequently expressed exasperation that foreign-born mothers willfully ignored their instructions, the wisdom that native-born practitioners dispensed sometimes reflected their own cultural tastes and preferences rather than purely scientific health care principles. They complained, for instance, that Eastern European mothers

insisted on feeding their children pickles, cooked cabbage, and other ethnic
foods which reformers themselves found repulsive, while Italian mothers allowed family members and even neighbors to lavish physical affection on
babies and small children, a custom that appeared disturbingly unhygienic
to many native-born health care workers. Alice Hamilton, a University of
Michigan-trained physician whose long career in Chicago health reform
included the supervision of a baby clinic in the basement of Hull House,
learned to be somewhat philosophical about this apparent cultural impasse.
"When I see the varied diet modern mothers give their babies, anything apparently from bacon to bananas," she commented in her 1943 autobiogra-
phy, "I realize that those Italian mothers knew what a baby needed far better
than my Ann Arbor professors did. I cannot feel I did any harm, however, for
my teachings had no effect." An apparent lack of foresight and planning on
the part of immigrant mothers served as another bone of contention between
reformers and their intended clientele. "Babies were fed whenever they
cried, frequently using up a whole day's feedings within a few hours," an
agent for the philanthropic McCormick Fund noted with impatience.[8]

Reformers were especially dismayed at immigrant women's habit of taking their children to visit neighbors afflicted with contagious diseases. Alice
Hamilton related the story of an Italian woman who lived in the neighborhood surrounding Hull House. Hamilton once chastised this woman for deliberately exposing her own children to contagion by taking them with her
when she entered a neighbor's house in order to nurse a family stricken by
diphtheria. "All sickness comes from God," the woman answered Hamilton.
"He sends it as He will." A *castiga*, or divine retribution, might be the dire
consequence if she had disobeyed the more important moral imperative that
women help each other in times of trouble: "He would rather send punish-
ment if I had not been kind." From this mother's own perspective, Hamilton
came to understand, the actions she had taken represented a calculated risk
rather than an act of careless negligence. (Hamilton also reported that the
children did not contract diphtheria after all.)[9]

For progressives who viewed health reform as a crucial means of acculturating the foreign-born into the American way of life, a necessary first step
was to change what they perceived to be a disturbingly fatalistic attitude toward illness and death widely held by new arrivals from southern and eastern
Europe. Such a transformation was essential, of course, if the modern notion
of *preventing* disease from striking in the first place was to take root within
immigrant communities. "Ignorant people have a curiously irresponsible
way of attributing all misadventures to Providence," Mary Aldis of the Chi-

cago Visiting Nurse Association (VNA) alleged in 1912. "Like an earthquake or a thunderstorm, they consider sickness as something beyond their control."[10] Such assessments are somewhat misleading, however, since native-born reformers' own perceptions of what actually constituted the physical states of being ill and being well may have differed markedly from those of their foreign-born neighbors.

By the early twentieth century, "good health" had for most urban, middle-class Americans come to mean a general sense of well-being and the ability to function at one's optimum level. Newly arrived European immigrants, on the other hand, were much more likely to define good health simply as the absence of any immediately life-threatening diseases. For generations of peasants from southern and eastern Europe, the performance of arduous physical labor remained crucial to survival, and therefore they placed a high cultural value on physical mobility; one was considered to be ill only at the point at which one became totally incapable of moving about.[11] Such starkly polarized definitions of health and sickness are well illustrated by the comment of one Chicago resident who recalled that "in Poland, people didn't talk much about illness, just dying. You were either healthy or you died." What reformers saw as their clients' extreme passivity or indifference toward illness was more likely a manifestation of immigrants' perception that, despite experiencing some undesirable symptoms, they already *were* in acceptably "good" health. As historian Roy Porter has observed, what has distressed patients throughout time is not their physical ailments per se, but rather the perception that illness is occurring contrary to their own expectations.[12]

Thus, in their self-proclaimed battle against immigrants' "fatalism" and "passivity" toward sickness and death, Progressive Era reformers ventured significantly beyond simply disseminating the fundamental rules of preventive health and hygiene among ethnic communities. They had also taken on the considerably more ambitious task of actually redefining for these communities what it meant to be in good health. Health reformers intended their campaigns to inculcate a new standard of physical well-being among their foreign-born neighbors, a higher set of criteria for determining what constituted an optimal state of health in twentieth-century America. Imparting a more enlightened set of definitions for health and illness was absolutely crucial, reformers believed, if Old World immigrants were to be successfully acculturated into a modern society such as the twentieth-century United States.

Because they accorded a central place to mothers' role in health care,

Chicago reformers deemed fatalism among foreign-born women to be especially deleterious to the welfare of immigrant communities. Many public health practitioners working in maternal and child health programs, for example, disparaged immigrant women as passive to the point of indifference regarding their own and their children's survival. But, contrary to reformers' perceptions, immigrant mothers had a number of solid cultural and psychological reasons to behave diligently in safeguarding their families' health. For immigrants from Italian, Jewish, and Slavic cultures, motherhood represented an exalted status, and women were socially and economically valued for the number of healthy children they bore and successfully raised. "A baby born back of the yards is a very common occurrence," commented Mary McDowell of the University of Chicago Settlement, "yet even when there are seventy-five in one block, each newcomer is loved and is an ever-new object of interest." Rearing a new generation in their adopted homeland provided an important sense of psychological continuity for foreign-born women now separated by long distances from their families of origin; losing their children represented a profound emotional loss.[13]

Immigrant mothers clearly were not indifferent to their children's well-being. But reformers and immigrants differed in their criteria for judging whether or not a specific case required the interventions of medical professionals. Although doctors were highly respected by European peasants, their expensive services customarily had been reserved for extreme emergencies rather than for routine ailments. One Polish man who migrated to Chicago, for example, remembered that mothers in Europe had fed their children tree bark as a cure for worms (a fairly common childhood affliction in agricultural regions), but his own parents had called in a physician when, at the age of three, he burned his hand by spilling lime on it. Once in the United States, immigrants continued the custom of calling upon medical doctors only after they had determined that the circumstances were serious enough to warrant such action.[14]

Seeking the services of medical professionals also entailed making difficult financial decisions, for the costs of such services could have catastrophic consequences for poor and working-class families. Contemporary family budget investigations by social scientists in Chicago demonstrated that Packingtown families commonly could not meet their minimum financial needs even under ordinary circumstances; the expenses incurred in cases of a severe illness or unexpected death could completely devastate a household budget. Further, a loss of household income due to illness or death frequently contributed to the impoverishment of families already living in economically marginal circumstances. In 1919 a report by the Illinois Health Insurance Commission identified sickness of a family member as an antecedent in up to one-half of all cases of impoverishment in the state; about one worker in five in this investigation had lost more than one week's employment due to illness.[15]

Immigrants' own recollections also reveal the ways in which a sudden illness or injury could severely disrupt their lives. A letter from a Polish man living in Chicago, for example, explained to his relatives still in Europe that his wife had been severely ill for ten weeks following childbirth, and the expense involved in her care had rendered him unable to send the steamship ticket he had earlier promised. Another woman recollected using her entire life savings of $250 to pay for the services of a physician when her mother was stricken with influenza in 1917 (despite receiving this medical attention, unfortunately, the woman's mother died).[16] In addition to cultural traditions concerning the use of professionals, then, economic considerations also clearly influenced immigrants' judgments regarding the most appropriate time at which to seek outside health care services.

It was a continual source of frustration to health reformers that mothers brought their children to local clinics only after they had become so ill as to be beyond medical help, even when health care services were being offered free of charge. In 1915, for example, public health nurses staffing a baby clinic in a Polish neighborhood commented that "the people here are most difficult to manage. They are mostly foreign born and are very suspicious of American methods." While some local mothers proved "quite amenable to reason," the nurses believed, others continued to harbor serious doubts about the safety of health care. "It was practically impossible to convince these mothers that sick babies were well cared for in hospitals," they complained. "Their babies are usually desperately ill before they are brought to us and quite frequently the unwilling mother, frantically clutching her baby in her arms, is literally dragged in by one of the public health nurses."[17]

Immigrant mothers actually had good reason to be wary of institutionalized medical care in early twentieth-century Chicago. Although charity hospitals had traditionally cared for indigent patients in cities throughout Europe, the quality of medical care that patients received in such institutions had been so appallingly poor that local residents had learned to turn to them only as a last, desperate measure — usually when the patient clearly had little or no chance for recovery. Maternal and infant mortality rates in urban charity hospitals in Europe were often frighteningly high. "In the old country no one ever was taken to the hospital unless as a very last resort, and the peasant watching the departing patient realized that he would be brought home to bury," asserted one contemporary observer of American immigrant life.[18] Nor were conditions necessarily better in the hospitals they encountered in their new homeland.

In the late nineteenth century, Chicago's public hospitals had earned a tarnished reputation for their exceedingly high mortality rates and had been avoided by all but the poorest native-born residents. Dr. Isaac Abt, a pioneer in the field of pediatric medicine, once recalled leaving Cook County Hospital over the weekend to find upon returning that every one of his little patients had died. As late as 1921, Caroline Hedger described the persistent belief she still encountered in her work among Chicago's ethnic communities that patients in Cook County Hospital were forced to drink from a "black bottle" in order to "finish" them. "How this belief arose I have never been able to find out," she confessed, "but I [have] heard it again and again." Hedger's exasperation reflected a widespread frustration among Chicago maternal and child health reformers that, despite their own vigorous efforts to dispel such grisly rumors, foreign-born mothers could not be persuaded to take their sick children to Cook County Hospital for much-needed medical attention.[19]

Immigrants' differing cultural sensibilities regarding illness, dying, and the appropriateness of professional care had prompted the founding of a number of hospitals in the late nineteenth century that were intended specifically to serve Chicago's ethnic communities. Jewish residents in the city, for example, established Michael Reese Memorial Hospital in 1882, while St. Mary of Nazareth Hospital had been founded in 1889 by Polish Catholics. The years between 1880 and 1902 saw a total of five new Catholic hospitals established to provide care to immigrant communities. In addition to medical services, religiously affiliated hospitals offered emotional and spiritual comforts that could not be duplicated within the secular environment of the city's public hospitals. In ethnic Catholic hospitals, as historian Christopher Kauffman has noted, the foods prepared, languages spoken, statues and holy pictures decorating the corridors, and the ministering of sacraments, all served as consoling reminders of the Old Country for immigrant patients, even transforming these hospitals into refuges from the anti-Catholicism and nativism immigrants experienced in their daily lives. A general distrust of secular medical institutions, combined with the considerable transportation and language difficulties they faced simply getting from place to place in a huge and often frighteningly confusing city, meant that Polish and Italian immigrants each made up only about 1 percent of all patients who were admitted to Cook County Hospital each year.[20]

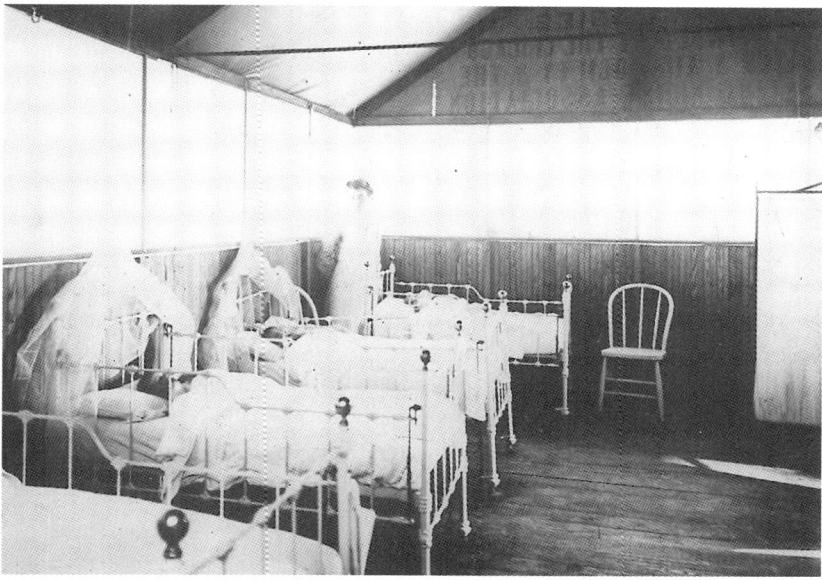

Figure 2.1. Visiting Nurse Association, interior of fresh air station for sick babies, Chicago, Illinois, 1910 (photographer unknown). Chicago Historical Society, photograph ICHi-03931.

Reformers hoping to eradicate untimely deaths due to infection or preventable diseases therefore were forced to find creative alternatives to traditional medical settings in order to woo immigrant mothers into seeking services for their children. More local — and thus more familiar — settings such as out-patient dispensaries, settlement houses, and neighborhood pure milk stations began to provide well-baby services such as the weighing and measuring of children to ensure that they were developing properly.[21] In the summer of 1905 the Chicago Relief and Aid Society, supported by the Chicago VNA, established the first of the outdoor baby tents that would prove to be extremely popular within the city's immigrant communities every summer for the next thirteen years (see figure 2.1). In establishing these innovative centers for children's health care, reformers responded as much to immigrant mothers' profound distrust of medical institutions as to their own conviction that tenement children chronically suffered from a lack of fresh air.

The first of these "small field hospitals" appeared on the roof of the Northwestern University Settlement at 1400 West Augusta, in the heart of a crowded Polish tenement district where the average family's weekly wage amounted to just ten dollars. The walls of the tent consisted of wooden boards three feet high with the remaining area screened to the roof. The roof itself was made of canvas with open spaces to admit light and air; the canvas was periodically sprinkled with water to keep the inside of the tent cool. Several iron cribs painted white, electric lights, electric fans, and a telephone furnished the interior.[22] Using the Northwestern Settlement tent as a model, the McCormick Fund established a number of similar outdoor tent clinics at settlement houses throughout the city. For several summers Hull House, for example, had a baby tent situated on its roof.

Health care personnel took great care to demystify any examination or therapeutic procedures they performed on their young patients, and neighborhood mothers were ensured full access to their children throughout their stay. "The mother could sit by and see all that the doctor did in his diagnosis, and she had the benefit of observing bathing and other care given by the nurse," Sherman Kingsley, the McCormick Fund's director, related. "Everything was in view, and if, when the child was ready for the tent, the mother did not yet have full confidence, she could sit down by the cot, and if it were a nursing baby, could return at intervals to feed it."[23]

After an initial period of mistrust, many immigrant women became active supporters of the baby tent program in their own neighborhoods. Health care workers reported with satisfaction that a number of mothers whose children had been cared for at the tents returned the following summer with their new babies. One Italian mother brought a new baby to her neighborhood tent each summer for three years. In one sad case, a woman apparently felt so confident of the care provided at the Northwestern University Settlement baby tent that she left her newborn infant with the nurses there and never returned; the settlement staff eventually located the mother, but the baby did not survive. During one ten-week period in the summer of 1913, seven tents posted throughout the city's poorest districts cared for a total of 1,260 sick babies. By 1917, staff nurses were pleased to note, mothers were bringing in babies "that were very slightly indisposed, whereas, four or five years ago, they waited until the babies were desperately sick before they would trust them to the tents."[24] Such reports from nurses and settlement workers on the front lines gave health reformers cause for optimism that their efforts to encourage among immigrant mothers a more active, enlightened approach to their children's health appeared to be succeeding.

But even after health reformers established a foothold in immigrant communities, neighborhood women continued to exert their influence by shaping institutional policies and practices. A 1914 publication from the McCormick Fund described the interactions between health care workers and neighborhood mothers as a "constant shuttle-like interplay . . . something usually lacking in the hospital regime."[25] When mothers visiting the University of Chicago Settlement's clinic balked at leaving their children there, health care workers came to realize that the iron cribs in which they placed children to sleep "presented to these people the appearance of a hospital and they became very suspicious of what the nurse was trying to do with their babies." Consequently, the staff replaced the iron cribs with hammocks that swung from the tent posts, and this arrangement apparently proved much more agreeable to neighborhood mothers. "There have been as many as fourteen of these hammocks at one time with babies in them," reported one investigator, "the mothers sitting around watching or fanning them and learning much from the nurse concerning the intelligent care of their infants."[26]

Even when immigrant women could bring themselves to entrust their precious babies to the care of health care workers, an overnight stay in the tents could prove especially traumatic for the mothers as well as the children. At one location, immigrant women made so many visits to check on their sick babies throughout the night that one staff nurse wondered if these anxious mothers ever slept at all. Repeated visits by the mothers throughout the night, sometimes with their sleepy older children in tow, eventually forced the baby tent operators to recognize and respond to mothers' own concerns by instituting an "official" policy of round-the-clock visiting hours. Health reformers learned to shape their programs and policies in response to local women's concerns, often formalizing changes that immigrant mothers, through their own actions, had already enacted.[27]

By 1915 representatives of maternal and child health agencies clearly were pleased at the apparent success of their efforts in reaching out to immigrant mothers. The Infant Welfare Society of Chicago, for example, was delighted to note that "one of the most pleasing features of the work has been the manner in which our mothers have been working with us and for us in spreading the propaganda and persuading friends to bring their babies to our conferences."[28] At the same time, however, most native-born health reformers remained either largely unaware or actively disapproving of the range of health care options already available to the immigrant mother within her own milieu. Ethnic communities retained their religious healing rites which often took place inside of private homes or on neighborhood streets — beyond the observation of outsiders to these communities. In addition, most reformers failed to recognize either the extent or the importance of immigrant women's informal networks for exchanging advice and volunteering services among themselves; they seemed rather unnerved, in fact, at the way in which immigrant women appeared to be frequently and casually entering into each others' homes.[29]

Immigrant mothers were not nearly as inert when faced with a child's sickness as health reformers tended to portray them in official reports. While medical professionals often interpreted local mothers' reluctance to utilize their own services as a sign of resistance to the *idea* of seeking medical care, it was really the proposed *methods* of curing that made these mothers skeptical. Unwilling to adopt unproven methods indiscriminately, immigrant women needed to be convinced that new therapeutic interventions being demonstrated really were effective before they decided to make use of them. Alice Hamilton's own experience at her Hull House health clinic enabled her to see this distinction clearly. She related the explanation offered by one Italian neighbor as to how one can know whether an illness was caused by a natural or a supernatural event. "You can tell easy," the woman reportedly told Hamilton. "If the doctor can cure you, it's a sickness. If he can't do nothing for you and the more medicine you take the worster you get, you're witched."[30] Like Hamilton's neighbor, most immigrant mothers believed they already knew the causes of their children's various illnesses, and therefore they decided when medical intervention was appropriate as well as the specific form of therapy required in any particular case.

One especially virulent threat to babies and small children was the Evil Eye, the power to willfully inflict harm or even death merely by looking at another person. Immigrants from southern and eastern European cultures believed that childless women possessing the Evil Eye employed it out of spite or envy, rendering mothers with beautiful and healthy babies particularly vulnerable to this malevolent force.[31] In the absence of bacteriological explanations for children's diarrheal diseases, the unseen power of the Evil Eye provided a compelling explanation for why a perfectly healthy and normal baby could suddenly fall ill, rapidly worsen, and perhaps even die. During the steaming summer months when thousands of babies and small children languished in Chicago's tenements, the Evil Eye must have seemed a formidable force indeed.

To guard against disaster, southern and eastern European immigrant women generally kept their infants indoors during their first few months of life, much to the dismay of preventive health reformers who constantly extolled the benefits of fresh air and sunshine for children's proper physical development. (Italian mothers also may have been shielding their little ones from the pernicious illnesses they believed could be carried by wind currents or drafts.) When they did venture outdoors, immigrant mothers took special — and, if circumstances seemed to warrant it, quite elaborate — precautions such as placing tiny crosses or special charms made of teeth, fish bones, or keys on their children's clothing. Contemporary observers noticed that Polish immigrants seemed especially careful not to appear to be staring at newborn babies in public places, lest they be suspected of intending harm to the little ones.[32] Immigrant mothers' extreme care in sheltering their babies from strangers and their diligent use of protective charms indicate that, far from being apathetic or indifferent toward their children's well-being, these women quite conscientiously practiced their own forms of preventive medicine, meticulously managing whatever physical and metaphysical variables they believed to be within their own control.

Although health reformers sometimes expressed disappointment that foreign-born women appeared to be clinging stubbornly to their Old Country superstitions, immigrant mothers adjusting their own health care practices to an unfamiliar environment were more apt to combine both old and new elements in ways that made sense to *them*. First- and second-generation Polish immigrant women, one study has demonstrated, did not immediately discard folk medicine but instead adapted their customary practices by replacing the natural ingredients they had found in Europe with manufactured ingredients they could readily purchase in America. Interestingly, the women in this study were just as likely to turn to scientific medicine if they believed it would be more effective than traditional remedies in any specific instance. Similarly, studies of health care practices in urban ethnic communities during more recent times have demonstrated that first- and second-generation immigrant women commonly combine old and new therapeutic regimens when caring for their own or their families' health, picking and choosing from among a range of options those treatments that seem the most likely to bring about the desired results.[33]

In addition to their own therapeutic interventions, immigrant women also sought care from a variety of formal and informal medical practitioners within their communities including medical doctors, pharmacists, midwives, relatives, and local women with special gifts for healing. Ethnic lodges or mutual benefit societies commonly pooled members' resources to employ a physician from within the immigrant community whose services could be sought by its members in case of a family member's illness or injury.[34] The European custom of using midwives to assist in childbirth remained a practical choice for immigrant women who had established their new homes in Chicago. Often locally known and respected women, midwives were familiar with the mother's language, customs, and beliefs, and charged considerably lower fees for providing more services than medical doctors did. Cultural proscriptions against allowing men to be present at a birth also influenced immigrant women's decisions to retain midwives.

In 1915 the Illinois State Board of Health reported that of 1,200 midwives officially registered throughout the state, over 900 practiced in Chicago alone. Registered and unregistered midwives attended over 45 percent of all births in the city, and a sizable proportion of these represented births to first- or second-generation immigrant mothers. A 1919 report by the Illinois Health Insurance Commission, for example, reported that a midwife was used as the sole practitioner in 70.8 percent of Bohemian, 69.1 percent of Polish, 59.3 percent of Lithuanian, and 56.2 percent of Italian confinements. Further, immigrant women commonly used the services of midwives along with those of medical doctors. Oral history interviews from Chicago suggest a typical pattern in which immigrants employed midwives for routine deliveries but the midwives themselves called in physicians if "the case didn't look right."[35]

Most immigrant women had already become quite familiar with the requirements of the birthing process before bearing their own children, having attended the births of nieces, nephews, younger siblings, and neighboring babies. A Polish woman in Chicago, for example, recalled attending her older sister's delivery and even cutting the cord and tying it with string. The experience proved helpful when this woman gave birth to her own baby, and she also made sure to watch the midwife carefully "so that I know how the next one be." Despite the unwavering approval midwives received within immigrant communities, Illinois health reformers often blamed unhygienic habits and a lack of formal medical training among midwives for the high rates of maternal and infant death found in immigrant communities. In addition, many Chicago health reformers often expressed dismay at midwives' apparent willingness to perform abortions for poor and working-class women.[36]

A series of statutes enacted by the Illinois General Assembly between 1896 and 1915 resulted in increased state supervision of midwifery. In 1908 a joint committee of the Chicago Medical Society and Hull House, chaired by Dr. Rudolph W. Holmes, launched a major investigation into midwifery practices in Chicago. Local physicians and health reform activists Alice Hamilton and Caroline Hedger also served on the committee. Investigators reported being "agreeably surprised" at the "cleanliness of both the homes and persons" of the majority of the 223 midwives in their study, a finding they explained by noting that these women were married to steady wage-earners and therefore midwifery represented a source of additional, rather than primary, household income. All but one of the midwives were literate, although 50 percent could read and write in their native languages only. The worst hygienic conditions, according to investigators, existed among immigrant Polish, Bohemian, and Italian midwives, and the report's conclusion recommended a much greater degree of state involvement in the training and supervision of these practitioners. Despite extensive efforts to regulate or eliminate their practice in the state of Illinois, midwives maintained their popularity with their immigrant clientele in Chicago until after the Second World War.[37]

Pharmacists represented another group of practitioners providing crucial health care services within immigrant communities. Many immigrants regarded apothecaries as learned individuals who not only spoke the language and understood the customs of the neighborhood but were also willing to listen patiently to the health complaints their customers brought to them, even keeping special chairs in their shops for this purpose. In addition, the medical advice they offered was usually extended free of charge. Newcomers to the city commonly relied on neighborhood druggists for trustworthy referrals to other local medical practitioners such as physicians and midwives.[38]

Some health reformers worried that the traditionally high status of the apothecary among European peasant communities made immigrants especially vulnerable to medical quackery in this country. They noticed, with some degree of alarm, that their foreign-born neighbors seemed to be replacing their Old World amulets and talismans with equally unsatisfactory bottles of American patent medicine. "Faith in medicines is only one door removed from faith in charms," declared one exasperated social worker. "Its importance [in immigrant communities] is distinctly out of focus." The Chicago Medical Society accused local druggists of preying on the ignorance of foreigners by advertising false cures and concoctions in their shop windows and distributing circulars touting quack remedies to their customers. In an interesting contrast to physicians' highly critical view of the immigrant pharmacist, the VNA of Chicago acknowledged and accepted the importance of the apothecary within immigrant communities, astutely setting up its bases of operation inside druggists' shops in order to establish an initial foothold within the local neighborhood.[39]

Women desiring information on preventive health care or the availability of local medical services could also turn to the pages of the foreign-language press. These newspapers, published by ethnic political, social, and religious organizations, featured informational columns that often included advice from medical professionals on matters of preventive health and hygiene; they also served as important propaganda for the health reform movement, providing publicity within non-English speaking communities for lectures, fairs, demonstrations, and other events taking place throughout Chicago. The Polish Women's Alliance, for example, published the *Glos Polek* (Voice of Polish Women), which regularly advised its female readers on practical ways to maintain their own and their families' health. Religious and ethnic leaders often actively encouraged immigrant women to utilize neighborhood clinics and to participate in local preventive health education programs. In 1917 *Narod Polski*, a publication of the Polish Roman Catholic Union, urged "all Polish mothers who have the cause of health and hygiene at heart" to attend infant hygiene lectures given in their native language by the city's Department of Public Health: "Listening to them attentively and understanding them will teach one to avoid many maladies of the infant stage and can save you many expenses, sorrow and misfortune." Failure to observe the appropriate sanitary rules, the newspaper admonished its readers, was all too often the cause of "unpleasant encounters with the Board of Health, not to speak of the harm inflicted on the health of the Poles." In 1919, *L'Italia* ran a feature story on the work of the Italian Medical Society for the Health of Italian Babies. The society's work was vital to the community, according to this account, because a significant number of Italian babies remained the unfortunate "victims of infectious diseases, irrational feeding, and neglected hygiene" — presumably because their mothers had been derelict in their duties. Foreign-language newspapers sometimes carried advice columns written by local physicians. The *Dziennik Chicagoski*, for example, ran a series of letters from a Polish doctor in 1897 warning mothers that the warm summer months were approaching and advising them on various ways to protect their infants from summer complaint.[40]

Immigrant mothers might also scan the pages of ethnic newspapers for advertisements describing personal and household hygiene products and the services of local health care practitioners. Although commercial advertising by professionals was a common practice in ethnic communities, it nevertheless greatly annoyed Chicago health reformers concerned about new arrivals' vulnerability to medical quackery. Immigrants, reformers contended, did not always understand that copy lauding the skills of a practitioner had been paid for by the advertiser himself. One study conducted in 1918 concluded that some foreign-language newspapers in Chicago were receiving as much as 20 percent of their revenues from announcements that had been placed by local charlatans. Even more disconcerting to reformers, perhaps, was this study's finding that a significant proportion of such commercial messages were "extravagant and lurid" and often accompanied by graphic photographs depicting the physical symptoms of disease in a gruesome manner.[41]

Some ethnic newspapers, however, took pains to disassociate their publications from this kind of cheap sensationalism. A 1905 editorial in *Saloniki*, for example, warned Chicago's Greek community to be on guard against medical impostors in the city, reminding its readers that "Greeks of today, like their ancient counterparts, value health and hygiene." The editors of a Slovak newspaper stipulated that they must grant prior approval to all advertising copy and advised that they would reject any announcements "that would harm our clean reputation and the readers of this newspaper." The *Greek Star* assured its readers that it catered to advertisers only "of the best kind."[42]

Finally, immigrant mothers in Progressive Era Chicago were likely to have at least one encounter with a public health nurse; Chicago, along with New York City, developed the nation's largest municipal nursing staff in the early twentieth century.[43] Most Progressive Era reformers, in fact, regarded the public health nurse to be the key medical professional within their own vision of health reform, especially the visiting nurses who took medical services and preventive health instruction directly into the homes of immigrant families throughout the city. Supported by private fund-raising efforts as well as outright cash donations from elite Chicago women, public health nurses provided assistance at either no cost or a minimal contribution from the families they served. In 1917, for example, 71 percent of the visits made by employees of the VNA were made at no charge to the patient. Further, the level of service to immigrant families went considerably beyond what would normally be expected of a physician or even a midwife.

Unlike traditional medical practice, which centered on the needs of the individual patient, visiting nurses regarded the entire family or household as their focus of care. Annual reports from the VNA reveal the extraordinary extent of nurses' involvement in their clients' lives. In the 1920s, for example, a local settlement house referred a visiting nurse to a maternity case in the neighborhood. During the course of her visit, the nurse not only cared for the mother and newborn baby, she also treated the mother's infected foot, bathed the father who was ill with a temperature of 104 degrees, secured hospital care and an ambulance for two other sick patients living in the house, and even sent for the local parish priest so that he could provide further assistance to the family.[44] In addition to this exceedingly energetic level

of caregiving, visiting nurses took upon themselves a host of nonmedical responsibilities as well, including finding employment for their clients, arrang-
ing for children to attend school, and setting up household budgets. Visiting
nurse employees even attended sessions of the local domestic court, "following up cases into their homes, putting the fear of the law in some of them,
referring others to agencies equipped to meet their needs." The VNA's training manual instructed its nurses to take a "bland and child-like interest in
everything, from the cleanliness of the refrigerator to the pay envelope of
the entire family."[45] Within the strikingly comprehensive notion of health
care the VNA promoted, virtually no aspect of immigrants' lives was to be
overlooked.

The visiting nurse was her role
as a preventive health care educator. "'Nursing,'" asserted Edna L. Foley,
superintendent of nurses for the association, "'does not always imply that we
do it, for in many homes the visiting nurses are the teachers while the family
does the care." Visiting nurses gave mothers instructions in child hygiene
and homemaking skills along with demonstrating proper home care procedures for the sick and injured. The VNA, in fact, regarded its "moral influence" in teaching the value of cleanliness and healthful living as the greatest
source of its own authority.[46]

The organization also recognized, however, that nurses could exert no
influence at all without first gaining the trust and cooperation of their immigrant clientele. They were trained to memorize information about the families in their care and record it only after they returned to their stations, since
filling out forms in the presence of immigrant clients seemed to make them
apprehensive and distrustful. "Respect racial and local traditions wherever
you can," the nurses' manual directed. "When these must be disregarded,
let the family see that this is for the patient's welfare, not for their or your
convenience." This all-important trust would only be earned, the VNA
stressed, when nurses successfully demonstrated that the methods they promoted really were effective in curing disease and maintaining health. Visiting nurses were even advised to give health care instructions in the kitchen
in the belief that their female patients would feel most comfortable in that
room of the house.[47]

The visiting nurse did her part in reducing high rates of maternal and
infant mortality in Chicago by applying "a steady pressure of advice and
instruction" on mothers living in poor and working-class neighborhoods
throughout the city. The prenatal care VNA nurses provided consisted
mostly of advising expectant mothers on how to prepare necessary items

such as clothing and infant feeding supplies for the impending delivery. The greater part of their maternity work was performed in the ten to fourteen days following a birth and included the personal care of the mother and infant as well as instructing her in postpartum and infant hygiene. Nurses calling on maternity cases in Chicago's poorest neighborhoods learned to bring clean baby gowns along with the other supplies in their medical bags since they frequently found their newborn patients wrapped in rags or even old newspapers.[48]

The VNA's conscientious efforts to earn the trust and cooperation of immigrant women paid off well, for the organization's annual reports reveal a striking increase in the number of visits made throughout the city each year. In 1890, its first full year of service, the association recorded a total of 8,586 visits; by 1917 this number had mushroomed to an impressive 241,352 visits. Their yearly caseload, according to the organization's own reckoning, brought visiting nurses in contact with "almost every nationality on the face of the globe . . . and every known disease." In 1911, for example, the greatest number of patients were identified as "American" (11,605), followed by "Polish" (3,601), "German" (2,038), "Colored" (1,741), and "Irish" (1,717). Of all the visits recorded that year, 1,929 represented maternity cases. The majority of these appeared to have been routine deliveries, but included among the problems nurses reported were 46 post-abortion complications, 136 miscarriages, 19 cases of puerperal septicemia, 3 puerperal hemorrhages, 24 "other diseases of parturition," and 51 cases of newborns requiring special feedings. Visiting nurses recounted that in addition to maternity care, their immigrant patients sought advice on everything from how to raise chickens in tenement buildings to whether a family member should stay in America or return to Europe. In one especially poignant account, grieving parents implored a nurse to baptize their baby when all hope for the little one's survival had been lost.[49]

The VNA's successful model of maternal and infant nursing care among immigrant communities, in fact, inspired a number of other organizations to establish visiting nurse services of their own. The Infant Welfare Society of Chicago, for example, hired nurses to visit with mothers in their homes to ensure they were following the infant care and feeding instructions given out at its well-baby stations. Originally established as milk distribution centers, the society's stations had quickly evolved into neighborhood health clinics where women brought their infants to be examined and weighed by volunteer medical personnel. Nurses then called on mothers and advised them in "all matters pertaining to the daily life of the baby: i.e., preparation of food, bathing, clothing, ventilation, etc." Like the VNA, the society remained mindful of the fact that, in providing information and advice on prenatal and well-baby care, it served the equally important function of acculturating immigrants to American norms and values concerning health. "The work of these visiting nurses," asserted F. S. Churchill, "is destined to be a weighty factor in the education, enlightenment, and assimilation of the great mass of our ignorant immigrants."

Some organizations attempted to facilitate the acculturation of Chicago's foreign-born residents by employing first- or second-generation immigrant women as nurses. The employment of ethnic nurses, these organizations hoped, would help to erode the barrier of language and cultural differences that stood between native-born reformers and immigrant communities. The VNA, for example, employed Bohemian and Polish women who were graduates of the Illinois Training School for Nurses; its annual report for 1915 includes a letter from a patient expressing "magnificent thanks" for sending a Polish nurse.[50] The Infant Welfare Society's first annual report brimmed with optimism about the work being performed by the ethnic nurse it had included on its medical staff:

> In the Polish section the mother looked rather dubious when she opened the door and saw the nurse. "Dzien dobre yak pan dziecko [Hello, how is your child?]" and her face would light up. Someone to talk to her in her own tongue about her baby! The nurse seldom fails to gain her confidence and so gradually the mothers are learning that the doctors and nurses are interested in each one of their babies, and they are coming to us full of confidence and faith in our judgment.[51]

Infant Welfare Society records demonstrate that, in addition to their medical competence, its visiting nurses were evaluated on their attitude, adaptability, and tact when dealing with their foreign-born clientele.[52]

Despite the agencies' apparent enthusiasm for the principle of using ethnic nurses to serve Chicago's immigrant communities, the actual number employed in public health work probably remained quite small. Relatively few women were likely to have had both the required proficiency in several different languages and the nursing training to meet licensing requirements in Illinois. Nursing historian Susan Reverby, in fact, has pointed out that the profession remained overwhelmingly dominated by native-born women until after the Second World War.[53] Interestingly, Caroline Hedger's assessment of the performance of ethnic nurses was actually rather negative.

Hedger had employed the services of ethnic nurses on several occasions in her own public health work among immigrant families in Packingtown. But in 1919, at a conference of the American Child Hygiene Association, she expressed displeasure that second-generation immigrant nurses tended to look with scorn upon their "greenhorn" clientele and often displayed an unreasonably sharp impatience with the continued practice of Old World customs by foreign-born women. Poor and working-class immigrant women, on the other hand, sometimes expressed skepticism or even hostility toward nurses from their own country because they assumed these educated, uniformed women originated from a superior social class and therefore actually disdained their clientele. Such intergenerational and class tensions, however, probably did not predominate in interactions between visiting nurses and immigrant communities since ethnic nurses represented only a small proportion of health care workers in Chicago.[54]

By contrast, enlisting nurses of color to provide health care to Chicago's black population met with considerably greater success. Members of the black community, in fact, frequently perceived nurses more favorably than they did physicians. As elsewhere in the nation, African Americans' access to professional medical services in Chicago remained severely restricted; the public health nurse practicing at a neighborhood clinic or visiting them in their homes appeared as the health care practitioner most responsive to their needs.[55] In 1905, after some discussion by its board of directors, the VNA hired Tallahassee Smith, a graduate of the Nurses' Training School at Chicago's Provident Hospital and one of the first nurses of color employed in public health work in the United States. In Chicago's racially segregated health care environment, Smith worked within the African American community almost exclusively; the VNA's annual reports, however, do record some apparent resistance from patients when Smith appeared at the homes of white Chicagoans. By 1920, the VNA had employed four black nurses who made a total of 15,088 visits to 3,615 patients in the city that year.[56]

Accessible, multiskilled, and extraordinarily dedicated to the well-being of their clients, public health nurses became the main links in the chain of educational programs and health care services forged by preventive health reformers in Progressive Era Chicago. Their work was not entirely without controversy, however. Many poor and working-class people understandably resented the seeming omnipresence of the visiting nurse in their homes and neighborhoods, finding her "child-like interest" in their family affairs rude and intrusive rather than helpful. To many immigrants from southern and eastern Europe, uniformed nurses may have appeared suspiciously more like unwelcome agents of the police than compassionate caregivers, an impression that undoubtedly was reinforced when nurses called in city officials to address some of the more egregious sanitary violations they encountered in ethnic neighborhoods. Mary McDowell cautioned nurses visiting Packingtown that "Slavs are a sensitive people, easily hurt by a gesture or laugh when they cannot understand the language."[57] In addition, Jewish and Catholic immigrants may have associated the native-born nurses arriving at their doorsteps with the "friendly visitors" from Protestant religious missions and thus regarded their underlying motives with misgiving.

Ultimately, however, it was another source of friction that would prove to be most detrimental to the development of public health nursing services in Chicago. Although visiting nurses regarded growing caseloads as proof of their success in gaining the trust and cooperation of their immigrant clientele, an increasing number of physicians in private practice saw public health nurses' expanding influence as an encroachment upon their own professional prerogatives. Nurses in public health practice quickly learned to be sensitive to doctors' concerns. When in 1909 the VNA joined forces with the United Charities and the Chicago Health Department in the campaign against childhood diarrhea, for example, project director Caroline Hedger reported with satisfaction that the nurses had made "a great effort to prevent friction with the medical profession."[58] In time, as preventive health education campaigns grew in visibility and influence in Chicago, the tensions between public health practitioners and private physicians would engender a major controversy that would spill over into the arena of Illinois state politics.

After building momentum for several decades, organized and systematic efforts to improve health in Chicago's immigrant communities received yet another major boost in the years during and immediately following the First World War when the imperative to acculturate immigrants took on all the proportions of a national crisis. While the Americanization of the immigrant had been central to the Progressive Era vision of social reform, the nation's official entry into the European war touched off a new — and decidedly more strident — emphasis on the need to do the job as quickly and efficiently as possible. Americanization emerged as a social reform movement in its own right during the First World War, albeit one with a number of differing sponsors and agendas.[59] Immigrant mothers, however, remained a central focus of concern, for native-born Americanizers perceived them to be primarily responsible for the transmission of cultural values within their families and communities. Further, many believed immigrant women had a strongly conservative influence on their families, clinging stubbornly and irrationally to the outmoded folkways of the Old Country, even when such beliefs and practices had become impractical — or even dangerous — within their new environments in the American industrial city.

Americanizers, in fact, often singled out immigrant women as *the* major obstacle impeding their acculturation efforts. The foreign mother, they asserted, remained isolated from the American way of life by the twin barriers of language and the Old World cultural traditions that kept women's activities confined primarily within the walls of their own homes. "She gets out of the home very little, far less than the husband," Dr. Michael M. Davis of the Boston Dispensary asserted during a round-table conference on the problems of foreign-born women held during the American Child Hygiene Association's 1918 annual meeting in Chicago. "She is burdened with the care of the husband and children and kept within a very narrow circle of duties most of the time. The isolation of the foreign mother carries with it problems we must wrestle with." Assigning the foreign-born mother an unparalleled degree of influence within the immigrant family, wartime Americanizers perceived a need to tailor many of their programs and policies to attract the participation of immigrant women specifically. Only if "the mothers of the family become Americanized," argued Gertrude Van Hoesen of the United States Department of Agriculture's Home Extension Service, "will the American standard of living which the father will learn at the factory and the children at the schools become a working plan in the family."[60] Wartime programs of accelerated Americanization, therefore, could only hope to succeed if they placed immigrant mothers at the very center of their operations.

The experience already gained by several female health and social welfare reformers in reaching out to Chicago's immigrant women put them into advantageous positions for assuming leadership roles in Americanization activities once the United States entered the war. Mary McDowell, for example, worked in coordination with the Chicago Board of Education to bring English language instruction to factory women in the workplace. Caroline Hedger chaired a special subcommittee on Americanization under the Woman's Committee of the Illinois Council of Defense. She also authored a pamphlet entitled "The Well Baby Primer" which utilized a child-care vocabulary to teach English to immigrant mothers. Published by the McCormick Fund, more than 3,000 copies were distributed throughout Chicago.[61] Like a number of native-born and middle-class women in this era, Hedger perceived such Americanization activities as an important new means for drawing immigrant mothers from southern and eastern European

cultures out from under what appeared to be an entirely subjugated existence in their tenement homes. These female reformers stressed that Americanization programs should be designed for the special benefit of immigrant
women — not their husbands, fathers, or sons. The immigrant mother was
the "victim of tyranny and oppression," Hedger asserted in an address before
the Child Welfare League of Peoria, "not only the tyranny and oppression
which governments and society have put upon the man, but added to these
the heavy, tyrannical hand of her husband." To Hedger, then, remaking the
immigrant mother into a modern American one also entailed liberating her
from the obsolete patriarchal dominance of Old World men. Sophonisba
Breckinridge of the Chicago School of Civics and Philanthropy took this
vision of emancipation one step further, proposing a restructuring of the nat-
uralization process so that a demonstrated proficiency in "fit motherhood"
qualified immigrant women to become American citizens independently of
their husbands' citizenship status.[62]

Wartime Americanizers took to unprecedented heights the progressive
stress on preventive health and hygiene education as a means of acculturating the foreign-born. Discussions on the topic of health reform among
immigrant communities virtually filled the pages of books, articles, and
conference proceedings produced by the Americanization movement, reaching their apex in the period just after the armistice. In 1919 Dr. Walter H.
Brown, for example, reading a paper on the "Health Problems of the
Foreign Born" before a meeting of the American Public Health Association,
appealed to his audience "to make a careful study of this matter in their own
communities and to insist that into any Americanization program shall be
incorporated a proper consideration of health." The ideal American citizen
was, among other things, a scrupulously clean and robustly healthy individual, and thus preventive health and hygiene instruction could not be
regarded as a trivial or auxiliary concern within the Americanization
movement. Good health, in fact, represented a core attribute of the modern
identity Chicago Americanizers were endeavoring to promote among their
city's citizens-in-the-making. "The good citizen works for public health," proclaimed a poster in a traveling exhibit from the National Child Welfare
League, further encouraging its onlookers to "fight disease by good personal habits."[63]

To Americanizers, the continued prevalence of sickness and untimely
death in many immigrant communities stood out as a conspicuous symbol
of the ignorance and backwardness that must be eradicated if the foreign-
born were to be successfully acculturated. "The numberless habits, customs,

standards, upon which personal and family hygiene are based," argued Michael Davis, "are everyday elements in determining the extent to which people are developing as Americans, members-in-full of an American community." Further, in this period of heightened patriotism and national pride, continued high rates of diseases that were known to be largely preventable if only proper care were exercised appeared not only un-American, but somehow even anti-American as well. If hygienic habits were known to save lives, Americanizers reasoned, then it became a matter of patriotic duty to practice them.[64]

Health reformers' model of modern motherhood represented an urban, middle-class domestic ideal that stood considerably removed from the reality of most immigrant women's lives. Speaking at a special conference on Americanization held under the auspices of the Department of the Interior in 1919, for example, Bessie A. Haasis of the National Organization for Public Health Nursing described the vital example that would be set for the immigrant community at large by those mothers who chose to adopt modern standards of hygiene during childbirth. Immigrant women, according to this account, could signal their successful assimilation into American society by choosing to engage the more modern services of a physician or visiting nurse rather than those of the more customary midwife. Haasis described an apocryphal scene in which "foreign neighbors" come to visit a new mother:

> Catching sight of the patient, now resting comfortably in a clean and tidy bed, with hair arranged neatly in two braids, by the side of her oval face, the baby asleep by her side, they exclaim, "Well, now you look like an American lady!" And does she not? And has she not learned what is the custom for American ladies in the way of comfort and cleanliness? And will she not know hereafter that this is her due as an "American lady," for at least 10 days after the baby is born, even though in the old country she might have been expected to get up and do her housework or go into the fields on the third or fourth day? . . . [The] mother and baby are started on the high road toward being Americans.[65]

Of course, this particular plan for transforming immigrant mothers into American ladies by altering their perinatal customs presupposed that such women were economically positioned to afford both the services of a medical professional and a respite from their own paid labor. Child welfare advocates had long voiced their concerns about possible hazards to infant health when mothers returned to work shortly after giving birth, including unsanitary bottle feeding practices and the potential negligence of surrogate caregivers. Further, the safeguarding of maternal and child health served as a fundamental guiding principle in the movement for protective labor legislation for female workers.[66] While all health reformers could agree that modern American motherhood required clean birthing rooms and an appropriate interval of rest for postpartum women, precisely how this goal could be achieved by mothers from all socioeconomic classes remained less than certain.

More radically inclined social welfare advocates proposed a system of maternity insurance that would compensate new mothers for the wages lost when they remained at home to care for their little ones; a number of countries, including Germany, Great Britain, and Russia, had experimented with such plans before the outbreak of hostilities in Europe.[67] But in the United States, where social support systems for the benefit of poor and working-class mothers had not been established, the "high road to being American ladies" more closely resembled a tightrope without a safety net. The First World War had thrown the goal of building a healthier citizenry into high relief. But, in the zeal for promoting hygienic motherhood that the nation's entry into war engendered, crucial questions concerning the role of the state in preventive health and maternal and infant care went virtually unaddressed. Remaking the Old World mother into a modern American one remained the focus of health reformers' concern.

3

Modernizing the Rural Mother

"What? Town Children Healthier Than Ours?" In 1927, the monthly magazine *The Farmer's Wife* expressed dismay at this revelation to its readership of some 750,000 rural women nationwide. Yes, Carroll Streeter's column went on to say, the evidence appeared to be unmistakable. Physical examinations of preschool-aged children in Illinois had revealed that rural children averaged 2.13 "significant defects," whereas those from the city averaged but 1.64. "For several years it has been increasingly apparent," commented one Illinois Department of Public Health official, "that the large cities are coming to be more healthful than the small communities and farming districts."[1] In the period from 1910 to 1930, rural periodicals like *The Farmer's Wife* acted as key players in a lively public discourse concerning the relative healthfulness of city versus country life.

Progressive Era health and child welfare advocates—for whom high rates of infant mortality served as yardsticks by which to measure society's overall state of advancement—had tended to portray the persistence of preventable disease and untimely death as a crisis of modern urban life, largely the result of waves of immigrants crowding into tenement neighborhoods and Old World mothers stubbornly clinging to their superstitious health care practices. But a startling reversal in the relative safety of urban and rural children was now becoming apparent. By the 1910s, urban infant mortality rates in the United States death registration area had declined rather dramatically while rural rates had either remained steady or dropped only slightly; by 1930, rural areas actually surpassed urban areas in recorded rates of infant death.

The health picture for Illinois children reflected the national trend. While in 1926 Chicago's infant mortality rate had fallen to 66.57 per 1,000 live births, the rate for the downstate region stood at 71.51. Health reformers

Table 3.1
Population of Illinois, 1890–1930

Year	Population	% Urban	% Rural
1890	3,826,352	44.9	55.1
1900	4,831,550	54.3	45.7
1910	5,638,591	61.7	38.3
1920	6,485,280	67.9	32.1
1930	7,630,654	73.9	26.1

Source: Clayton, The Illinois Fact Book and Historical Almanac, 1673–1968 (1970), p. 38.

credited preventive health and hygiene campaigns for the urban success story. "The reduction in infant mortality which has taken place in cities," asserted the United States Public Health Service, "has probably been due largely to increasing emphasis being placed on the principles of sanitation, to the establishment of well-baby clinics, to increasing use of hospitals for delivery, to compulsory pasteurization of milk, and to the application of modern medical knowledge."[2]

The intractability of high maternal and infant death rates in an age of modern, scientific health and hygiene practices connoted a certain backwardness and even ignorance among the rural population, a disagreeable state of affairs that prompted numerous discussions in agricultural magazines, especially those aimed at a female audience. Farm babies should be healthier than their town cousins, asserted The Farmer's Wife, because of the advantages posed by "heaven's sunshine and the fresh, pure air." Unfortunately, it was becoming increasingly evident that this was not the case, and, in fact, city children appeared to be the healthier group. "Since we are obliged to admit this," The Farmer's Wife continued with a hint of chagrin, "we should know why these apparently favorable circumstances are not working, in all cases, to the advantage of our country children."[3]

While health reformers' rhetoric set up a dichotomy between the healthfulness of town and country, clear disparities among rural dwellers themselves shaped public health conditions in important ways. Although historians have characterized the period from 1900 to 1920 as a "golden era" in American agriculture, the prosperity of these years did not touch all rural dwellers equally. The rural population of Illinois was declining (table 3.1). Throughout the midwestern grain belt, the high cost of newly available farm machinery was driving many smaller and less productive farmers off the land. The period from 1900 to 1920, in fact, saw a 500 percent increase in the total dollar value of mechanical farm implements in use throughout the state of Illinois. Unable to invest the large amount of capital required to purchase the new machinery, smaller producers were forced to give up their land, frequently to the benefit of wealthier farmers. While the average size of individual farms in the state increased, the total number of farms in the state actually decreased. In 1900, for instance, 264,151 individual farms existed in Illinois; this number was reduced to 250,853 by 1912, a decrease of 5 percent. The downward trend continued, so that by 1930 only 214,497 farms remained in the state, a decline of over 18 percent since the turn of the century. The growing reliance on technology also meant that fewer human hands were needed to perform more traditional chores in the field. Many of those who could neither own their own farms nor find work as hired agricultural laborers eventually migrated to Chicago.[4]

Concentration of farmland ownership into fewer and fewer hands strengthened the practice of tenant farming in Illinois. Tenant farms had represented 39 percent of all farms in the state in 1900, but this proportion rose to 43 percent by 1930. One contemporary survey put the proportion of tenant farms in Illinois even higher, at nearly 53 percent. Rates of farm tenancy tended to be higher in those regions within the state where the farmland was more valuable. Although tenant farming often represented only a temporary status for midwestern families (many young farmers, for instance, rented land while they waited to either purchase or inherit their own farms), nevertheless some urban-based health and social welfare reformers in the Midwest expressed alarm at its spread throughout the region, influenced no doubt by the highly negative social stigma that had come to be associated with this practice in the South.

A pattern of socioeconomic stratification that served to differentiate the state's northern from its southern counties — developments strongly evident since the mid-nineteenth century — actually became more pronounced during the first decades of the twentieth century. Farmers in the northern portion of Illinois tended to be more prosperous, their land more productive and more valuable, and their material circumstances distinctively advantageous in comparison with those in the state's southern region. The relatively poor soil of southern Illinois rendered that region unsuitable for growing major cash crops such as wheat and corn, commodities that were becoming an increasingly important staple of midwestern agriculture in this period. Southern Illinois farmers, therefore, were turning instead to the less profitable business of orchard farming. Agricultural census data for 1920, for example, reveal that the average dollar value per acre for farms in the twenty counties at the state's northern end ranged from $135.62 (McHenry) to $262.49 (La-Salle), while for the twenty counties at the state's southern end this measure ranged from $23.74 (Pope) to $111.19 (Wabash).[5]

The unevenness of rural economic development in this period was reflected quite markedly in the varying material conditions to be found within farm homes. In 1915 the Household Science Department of the University of Illinois undertook a major survey of the material circumstances of farm families throughout the state. The survey, covering 38,000 homes (nearly 12% of all farm households in Illinois), revealed that northern Illinois farm families enjoyed relatively larger and better-equipped homes. While the vast majority of all Illinois farm homes were still heated by stoves, for example, 6.6 percent of northern homes but only 1 percent of southern homes were equipped with hot-air furnaces. Hot water tanks had been installed in 8 percent of northern but only 5 percent of southern farm homes, while indoor toilets could be found in 10.4 percent of northern but only 2 percent of southern farm homes; less than 4 percent of southern homes were equipped with facilities for a shower-bath. Fully 59 percent of the southern farm families surveyed in 1915 drank water that had been obtained from open or uncovered wells. Illinois public health reformers were interested but not surprised to discover that the incidence of typhoid fever in the state followed the same basic geographic pattern as the distribution of indoor plumbing facilities installed in rural homes; death rates from typhoid fever were in fact significantly lower in northern than in southern counties.[6]

African Americans, who historically had represented only a small minority of Illinois farmers, saw their numbers decline even further during the early twentieth century, from 1,486 in 1900 to just 893 in 1920. Although the black population of Illinois nearly quadrupled between 1900 and 1930, almost three-fourths of the state's African American citizens lived in Chicago. Lack of capital as well as white prejudice in lending money and renting land meant that only a small proportion of blacks remained farmers in Illinois. The vast majority of African Americans who stayed on the land could be found in the state's southernmost counties, where the land was less productive and therefore less expensive. Census data for 1920, for example, reveal that of the state's 893 black farmers, more than 70 percent lived in the southern one-third of the state; slightly more than 26 percent resided in Pulaski County alone, a county situated along the border with Kentucky. Much of this land remained largely unimproved since Charles Dickens had published his scathing descriptions of the region in 1842. Some 220,000 acres in eight counties at the southern tip of Illinois were composed of undrained swampland; as late as 1914, state public health officials recorded more than fifteen malarial deaths per year in each of these counties.[7]

In the pages of social reform and progressive farm journals, in papers delivered at public health conferences, and in numerous published surveys of rural communities, farm women and their babies were portrayed as the primary victims of the unsanitary, unventilated, and disease-ridden conditions of country life. "The problem of the farm woman," declared the *Literary Digest* in 1920, "finally has assumed proportions sufficiently alarming to call forth . . . a note of warning to the country." Surveys conducted by the U.S. Department of Agriculture (USDA) and the Children's Bureau led some reformers to conclude that infant mortality rates in rural areas were becoming so distressingly high that they were actually driving young women away from the family farm. Few girls contemplating their futures as wives and mothers, they concluded, would choose to remain on the farm where "child life is at a premium. . . . The farmer's wife too often sees the cradle emptied for the grave." Progressives found this prospect especially upsetting because farm women represented the very foundation of the rural family, and family life was in turn the foundation of agrarian society.[8]

Indeed, to some activists in progressive reform circles, rural life itself seemed to be in imminent danger of collapse. Country dwellers were defecting to the cities in droves, and many urban-based reformers interpreted this mass exodus, not as a reflection of the changing agricultural economy, but rather as the result of a marked deterioration in the quality of agrarian life. The dazzling array of amenities being introduced into the modern urban middle-class lifestyle in this era — innovations such as labor-saving technologies for the home, more reliable and liberating modes of transportation, and the glamour of popular entertainments such as motion pictures — had made the simple pleasures of country life seem dull and backward by comparison. Unpaved and frequently impassable roads, houses lacking electricity and indoor plumbing, and a dearth of cultural and educational opportunities inspired little motivation, reformers argued, for the younger generation to remain on the farm. The wretched health conditions which many country mothers and their children endured seemed to be yet another dismal fact of rural life, lending a new urgency to the discomfiting message of agrarianism's inexorable decline.

Such anxieties had prompted the formation of the Country Life Movement — the "rural arm of progressivism" — whose adherents aimed to preserve the agrarian way of life by transforming rural dwellers into more efficient, productive, and modern citizens. The movement was led by professionals from land grant colleges, government agriculture departments, and the rural press as well as from school, church, and social reform associations; the majority of the movement's adherents hailed from the Midwest. In 1908, President Theodore Roosevelt appointed a Commission on Country Life, chaired by Liberty Hyde Bailey, an agriculturalist at Cornell University. The commission's 1909 report chronicling rural social problems and offering suggestions for their solutions received a great deal of publicity and comment in both urban and rural venues.[9] From the beginning, the improvement of rural health conditions constituted a key item on the Country Life Movement's agenda. In 1919, for example, the American Country Life Association devoted its national conference exclusively to the issue of rural health reform. "It is evident," claimed George E. Vincent, president of the Rockefeller Foundation, "that the general movement for better and more satisfying living conditions in the country will more and more include hygiene, sanitation, and the promotion of health."[10] Country life advocates argued that organized and systematic campaigns on behalf of rural dwellers' health — modeled on the activities that had been underway for decades in urban areas — were crucial if the quality of agrarian life was to be satisfactorily "uplifted."

Like their progressive colleagues championing health and social welfare campaigns in the city, those who turned their attentions to rural health conditions in the early twentieth century acknowledged women as being primarily responsible for safeguarding both the emotional and physical well-being of their families and communities. "The health of the world must always lie in the hands of women," Julia Lathrop, chief of the Children's Bureau, told a female audience attending the 1917 Illinois Farmers' Institute, "and women must be trained for it."[11] Like their city sisters, then, country mothers were uniquely suited to advance the cause of rural uplift through their traditional obligations in maintaining cleanliness and order on the family farm. Further, because they were geographically isolated, country dwellers had a long history of relying on self-help for dealing with accidents and disease, and rural mothers traditionally had acted as their family's primary medical practitioner. "The people did not call on 'Old Doc,' the family practitioner, unless there was a serious accident or a life-threatening illness," a physician from central Illinois recalled in his memoirs. "They relied instead on home remedies to take care of their health needs."[12]

Such a characterization is corroborated by oral histories of rural Illinois residents who assert that physicians were rarely called in cases of moderate illness or minor accidents. Household guides such as the *Practical Farmer* recommended a well-stocked medicine chest and a book of instructions as necessities for every rural wife and mother. In 1919, the *Literary Digest* reported one survey's finding that farm wives spent an average of thirty days per year nursing the illnesses of family members. An observer of rural life in Illinois declared that "on the farm the mother of the house is the health department."[13] Ideally, then, the modern farm mother — like the immigrant mother in America's cities — would come to resemble more closely the urban middle-class mother in the definition and conduct of her womanly duties. The farm woman's obligation to ensure her family's physical well-being now must be updated and extended to include activities designed to safeguard the quality of agrarian life. The time had come, in other words, for rural motherhood to be recognized as an important public, as well as private, vocation. Juliet Lita Bane, a domestic economist conducting research for an M. A. thesis at the University of Chicago, concluded that while rural people must be urged to utilize whatever public health facilities were available to them, "A great deal of responsibility will rest upon the housewife and there are certain facts that she should know and certain principles that she should observe in safeguarding herself and her family against ill health and contagious diseases. She should have time to acquaint herself with the information necessary to do her part well."[14]

Bane's use of the word "housewife" is noteworthy because it reveals an important underlying tenet of rural health reform campaigns in the early twentieth century. Traditionally, of course, farm women did not experience the "separation of spheres" between the work and home environments which had come to characterize the urban middle classes since the previous century. For farmers, home and field remained equally essential bases for economic production long after the home had become the privatized shrine of urban middle-class family life. City-based reformers worried that farm women, engaged as they were in endless rounds of productive and reproductive labor, simply lacked adequate time to devote to the serious study of scientific motherhood. Acquiring knowledge about the latest preventive health care methods and the most up-to-date household hygiene techniques — and putting that knowledge to use not only for the betterment of her own family but for the neighborhood and community as well — would exact stringent new demands on the modern farm mother's time and resources. Women's productive burdens, therefore, must be alleviated in order to allow them to fully participate in the uplift of rural life. "It is poor business from every

standpoint," declared the U.S. Department of Agriculture's Florence E.
Ward, "if work out of doors means overstrained nerves and muscles resulting
from an attempt to take on these duties without releasing any household
tasks, or if it means neglect of housework or sacrificing attention to children,
with a consequent lowering rather than raising of the standard of living."[15]
For reformers, then, an essential element in the improvement of rural health
conditions was the necessity of overhauling women's place in agricultural
production so that her energies could be more fruitfully directed toward the
obligations of modern motherhood. The farm mother's responsibility for the
protection of her family's health, although traditionally an important feature
of the rural domestic economy, received a new emphasis as well as an elevated importance within rural public health campaigns predicated on a
vision of a modernized farm family.

But the serious study and intelligent implementation of new hygienic
theories and methods required an investment of time and resources that remained largely beyond the reach of a great many rural mothers. Beneath
the distinctly gendered discourse of rural health reform, then, lay a subtext
suffused with the precepts of social and economic class. The leadership role
being advanced for farm mothers within the rural preventive health campaigns that emerged in this period paralleled the one already carved out by
middle-class and elite women in cities such as Chicago. Despite health reform advocates' tendency to speak in terms of enlisting *all* country dwellers
in the cause of improving rural health standards, their progressive modernization rhetoric was more precisely targeted toward an emerging cadre of
women from relatively prosperous families in small towns and rural areas.
The preventive health and hygiene movement in downstate Illinois attempted to build a bridge between the health and social welfare activism
already exhibited by club women in Chicago and those rural women whose
time and resources conceivably could be freed sufficiently to allow them to
engage in public campaigns.[16]

Women who lived in the expanding ranks of tenant farming families
posed an especially vexing problem to Illinois health reformers. Since tenant
farmers did not own the land they worked, many reformers argued, they had
less of a stake in the betterment of rural life; they were, in the words of
one rural health advocate, "non-conductors of the currents of community
spirit."[17] Chicago public health nurse Katherine Olmsted, for example, argued that "we must recognize that a large per cent of the tenants are as a
rule a poor class, in debt up to their ears for horses, groceries, seeds, implements, fence wire and the doctor, and that the children are kept out

of school months at a time to help with the work. The wife and mother often ranks in intelligence with our foreign mothers in the cities."[18] The tenant farmer's ostensible lack of commitment, rural health advocates feared, would extend to a lax and indifferent attitude on the part of the farm mother regarding hygiene standards for the home and sanitary standards for the rural community at large.

The farm press became one of the most important vehicles for stirring up interest in preventive health and hygiene campaigns among middle-class farm women. During the previous century, farmers isolated from urban political and economic centers had come to rely heavily on journals and newspapers to keep abreast of the latest developments in agricultural methods and governmental policies, and farm households commonly subscribed to several such periodicals. The *Prairie Farmer*, for example, had served as one of the most influential farm periodicals in Illinois since its inception in 1841. The woman on the farm had also depended on the information presented in agricultural newspapers and journals, counting them "among her valued aids." By the early twentieth century, the overwhelming majority of midwestern farm women could read, and magazines written specifically for a female audience enjoyed widespread circulations throughout the region. Census data for 1910, for example, show that only 2.0 percent of rural adult females in Illinois were illiterate, as compared to 3.7 percent of the general adult population of the state. The 1915 University of Illinois survey had revealed that 68 percent of Illinois farm households subscribed to a weekly newspaper, while 68 percent took at least one farm journal, and 54 percent also received a popular ladies' magazine.[19]

Preventive health care became a mainstay of publications aimed at rural audiences in the early twentieth century. Articles offering advice on the hygiene of pregnancy and infancy proved to be an especially popular feature among the rural female readership, and by the 1910s most farm periodicals carried these items regularly. The Department of Hygiene and Public Health at the University of Illinois at Urbana-Champaign produced the *Health Advisor*, a weekly compendium of items on preventive health and sanitation topics that was distributed to newspapers throughout the downstate region.[20] Many publications invited mothers to submit directly their own questions concerning preventive health care. The advice columns of progressive farm journals, written for a readership of relatively well-to-do farm women, encouraged an informed approach to motherhood and suggested an elevated status for the farm woman's traditional responsibilities toward her family's well-being. Affronted by statistics implying that high rates of disease and death from preventable causes still existed in her own midst, the progressive farm woman as presented in magazines such as *The Farmer's Wife* actively sought to keep abreast of the latest information on hygiene, sanitation, and child care. Progressive farm journals regularly extolled the virtues of the "wide-awake" farm woman, whose vigorous efforts to keep informed and up-to-date about all aspects of farm and farm home management clearly distinguished her from her poorer and less educated sisters whose lives remained fettered by their own backwardness.

The guidance proffered in farm periodicals, whether by a physician, advice columnist, or editor, usually reflected contemporary sensibilities among preventive health reformers concerning the inherent value of fresh air and sunshine as well as the growing awareness of the role played by bacteria carried by water, milk, or flies, in spreading disease. "Fresh air is as important to the restoration of the child's health as the proper food," asserted the *Illinois Farmer and Farmers' Call*. "Keep the rooms free from garbage, soiled clothes, piles of newspapers that accumulate and retain dust, and from rubbish of every kind. The windows should be open day and night." In 1915 the editor of *The Farm Home*, a Springfield periodical, announced that child hygiene would now be included as a regular feature of the magazine's Mother's Department. "The babies of Illinois have not received due attention at the hands of editors," Charles F. Mills confessed to his readers. Mills invited mothers to send in photographs of their babies, and he selected pictures exemplifying the successful outcomes of proper child hygiene techniques to publish in subsequent issues.[21] The new child care column, edited by Mrs. Chelsea A. Tobin, included information on the normal growth of the baby, precautions for bottle feeding ("cooking" water, for example, to ensure sterilization), weaning, recording the child's birth, the dangers of elixirs and "soothing syrups" (which often contained narcotics or alcohol), and the proper accessories for furnishing a nursery.

The peril posed by disease-carrying flies played as a constant, ominous theme in advice columns read by Illinois farm mothers. "Is the fly dangerous?" the *Illinois Farmer and Farmers' Call* asked rhetorically. "He is man's worst pest and more dangerous than wild beasts or rattlesnakes." The fly, perennially portrayed as Evil Incarnate in farm women's magazines, stood accused of carrying diseases such as typhoid fever, tuberculosis, and summer complaint "on his wings and his hairy feet." "He may call on you next," warned one columnist in "The Fly Catechism": "Where is the fly born? In manure and filth. Where does the fly live? In every kind of filth. Is anything too filthy for the fly to eat? No. . . . How shall we kill the fly? Kill the fly in any way, but kill the fly."[22]

As medical historian Naomi Rogers has pointed out, the association between dirt, flies, and disease, although not always scientifically valid, nevertheless so compellingly combined morality with science that by the early twentieth century it had become a crucial cultural signpost for distinguishing "rich from poor, native-born from immigrant, the ignorant and careless from the informed and responsible."[23] Rogers's observation helps us to understand the vehemence with which flies came under attack in the magazines and newspapers written for an audience of middle-class farm women (figure 3.1). Although they were an inevitable presence in agrarian life, in the wake of the energetic rural public health reform efforts that were launched in this era, flies had now become a potent symbol of a farm mother's inexcusable negligence. The presence of flies in the farm home could no longer be tolerated, particularly by those women who were becoming increasingly sensitive to critiques about the apparent backwardness of country life. "One mother did not believe a little fly could hurt her young," *The Farmers' Wife* intoned dramatically in 1914. "One by one she laid away her babies until now they are three silent empty places in her heart."[24]

Farm women's journals were often unequivocal in their condemnation of unenlightened and slovenly country mothers. One woman's column editor proclaimed that millions of innocent children were being killed by their own mothers "because they are steeped in ignorance, and will not take the trouble to inform themselves concerning proper methods of child rearing." A mother's failure to educate herself about proper child hygiene measures, the columnist admonished, constituted nothing short of criminal negligence as, "in this day and age there is no excuse for such ignorance."[25] In contrast to her sleepy-headed and careless sister, the wide-awake farm mother dutifully screened windows, poured lime into privy vaults, and slaughtered untold numbers of flies with the paddles, sticky paper, kerosene oil, and insecticide powders advertised regularly in the pages of farm journals.

For those Illinois farm families who found themselves prospering in the 1910s and 1920s, it was increasingly becoming possible to "modernize" the farm home by purchasing the latest household technologies and consumer goods. Guaranteeing a sanitary and healthful environment in which to care for their families meant that farm mothers needed to acquire, among other things, indoor plumbing for their homes, sufficient supplies of clean water and milk, and access to the most up-to-date information concerning preventive health and hygiene. In 1913 the United States Department of Agriculture undertook a major survey with the aim of documenting and understanding farm women's working and living conditions. The survey, administered to women in families participating in agricultural extension programs, revealed

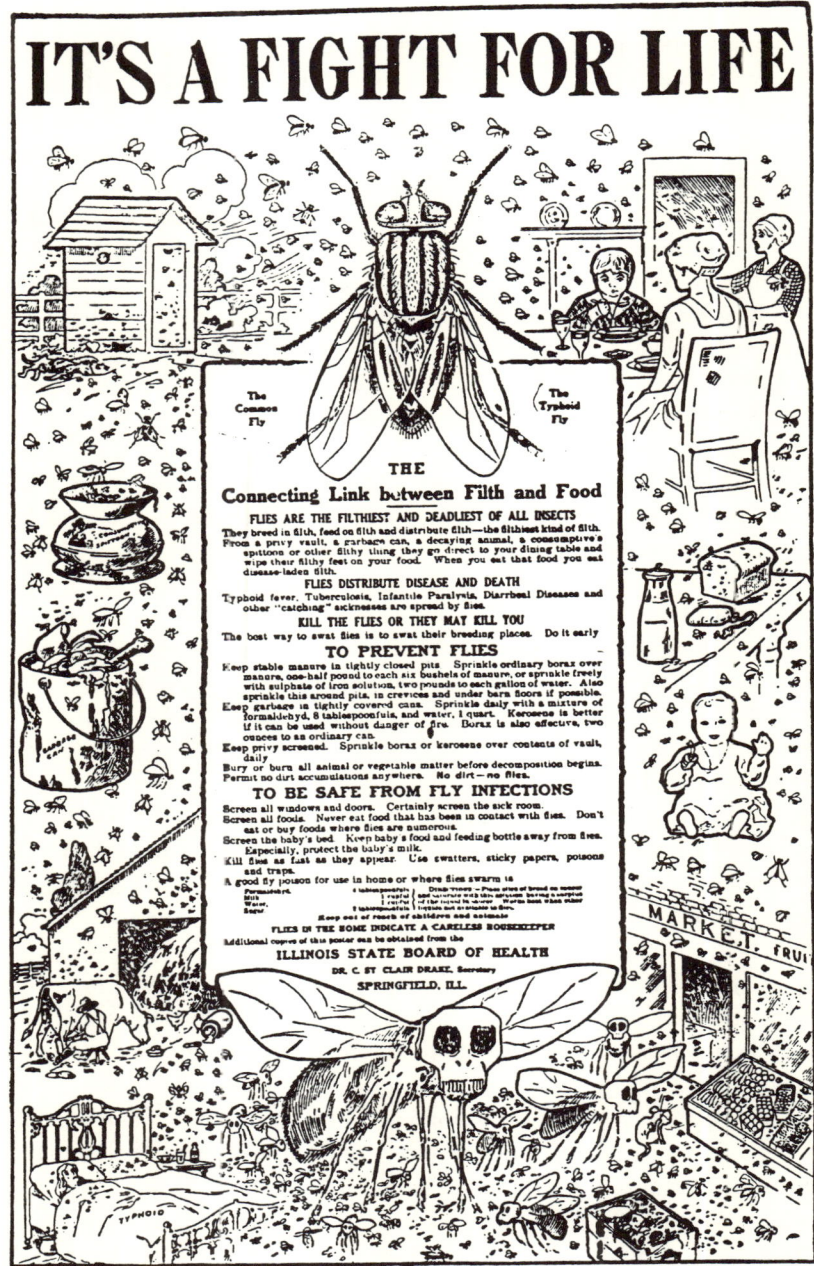

Figure 3.1. Illinois State Board of Health warning about the health dangers posed by flies, including the admonition, "Flies in the home indicate a careless housekeeper." *Illinois Health News*, March 1915.

that a foremost complaint for this group of farm women was the lack of plumbing in their homes. Respondents expressed these grievances primarily in terms of a desire to reduce their intolerably heavy workloads; many women complained, for instance, that the location of water wells on their farms had been determined for the convenience of the livestock rather than their own work needs, forcing the women to haul water several hundred yards daily. Perhaps even more significantly, responses from these relatively affluent farm women also demonstrated their own sense of *entitlement* to the benefits of modern technologies that were already widely available in the homes of their urban middle-class counterparts. "There's no farm wife who doesn't work hard enough to deserve the last notch in modern conveniences," one Illinois farm woman declared in a letter to *The Farmer's Wife*. Asserting that the acquisition of household technologies represented a matter of basic self-respect, this woman defiantly signed herself "I Won't Be a Hick." But if convenience emerged as a salient issue in the USDA survey, the improvement of the farm family's health represented an equally significant concern. The farm women who responded to this survey also demonstrated a growing awareness of the potential health hazards posed by outdoor privies, shallow wells, and uncovered cisterns, and they expressed a strong desire to improve health conditions within their own homes and communities. The USDA survey found that these farm women deplored the lack of *information* — as well as technology and household conveniences — that was available to them for ensuring that preventive health and hygiene measures could be carried out with appropriate diligence.[26]

But, even if farm women aspired to attain higher standards of cleanliness and sanitation in their homes, the patriarchal economic arrangements of American farming meant that the resources for acquiring the necessary commodities to effect such changes remained almost exclusively under the control of their husbands. As historian Katherine Jellison has demonstrated, this discrepancy did not go unnoticed by farm women themselves. In conveying their desire for modern technologies such as indoor plumbing, electrification, and the latest in household appliances, the USDA survey respondents were also challenging the unequal status that farm women continued to endure within their own households. Many women expressed resentment toward the disproportionate share of attention being given (by the government as well as by their husbands) to the modernization of agricultural production while the crucial work of human reproduction remained in the Dark Ages. They complained that their husbands were willing to purchase modern equipment for the field but balked at investing money in

indoor plumbing or electricity for the home. "For a number of years," one
Illinois farm wife protested, "the average farmer has had his county soil expert and crop advisor, cow testing association and so forth, with all the latest
inventions in farming apparatus . . . while the farmer's wife, in the majority
of cases is plodding on in the same old way her mother did before her."[27]

Overwork itself was often cited as a chief cause of the poor health plaguing farm women, and those corresponding with agricultural journals frequently decried the plight of the overworked–and largely undervalued–farm
wife. In 1915 the *Journal of Home Economics* reported one study's finding
that farm women in Illinois and Indiana worked an average of thirteen hours
per day year-round, including Sundays. The women's labor included the
preparation of meals, care of the house, sewing, laundry, marketing, caring
for children, poultry and dairy work, orchard and yard work, and procuring
farm and household supplies. "Care of the sick," an item not included originally in the survey's list of chores, apparently constituted a substantial part
of the farm woman's workload, for the respondents themselves wrote in this
item. As late as 1929, when the standard industrial work week had been reduced to forty-two hours, farm women still worked an average of sixty-three
hours per week.[28]

Although rural health reform advocates presumed to speak on behalf of
country mothers, farm women themselves, acutely aware of the enormity of
their workload, were not averse to voicing their own complaints. Mrs. Fannie
Tilton of Hoopeston proclaimed before a country women's club that, while
the annual Chautauqua remained of immense value in "bringing a bit of
pleasure into the sordid lives of us farm women . . . we want a little recreation oftener than once a year." One anonymous woman writing in *Wallace's
Farmer* applauded the idea of vacation camps for farm women which had
recently been established in Iowa and Illinois ("No Husbands, No Children,
No Dishwashing or Chickens for One Glorious Week"). A Champaign
County magazine claimed that one farm wife had actually calculated the
total cash value of her work to be $61,630.55, a sum exceeding the entire real
estate value of her farm. "If a reasonable commercial value were placed on
the work of the women and children on the farm," the *Banker-Farmer* declared, "it would equal in dollars and cents the total real estate value of our
nation." The *Literary Digest* facetiously suggested that farm women stage a
strike to protest their hours and working conditions.[29]

The subject of the potential damage to farm women's health posed by
overwork and exhaustion was not always treated so lightheartedly, however.
Farm women's grievances also reached the federal Children's Bureau in

Washington, D.C., through its extensive correspondence program. Many rural women's letters requesting advice in preparing for childbirth and the hygiene of pregnancy and infancy reflected conditions so distressing that they inspired the Children's Bureau to launch a series of studies of maternal health in rural communities. Anecdotal evidence gathered from these studies led bureau officials to conclude that rural women's geographic isolation and heavy physical workload were to a considerable extent contributing factors to continued high rates of maternal and infant mortality. While women residing in sparsely populated and geographically remote areas in the mountain states and high plains were clearly most at risk, even the relatively prosperous farm women represented in the bureau's Kansas study received very little prenatal care.[30]

In 1917, at the seventh annual meeting of the American Association for Study and Prevention of Infant Mortality, Dr. Grace L. Meigs of the Children's Bureau told her audience that rural women frequently expressed bitterness that the advice the bureau offered could not be carried out because the nearest doctor was too far away; the high cost of prenatal care also remained out of reach for the average farm family. "There is in several letters," Meigs commented, "a note of complaint that the Government in cases of hog cholera or other animal diseases stands ready to help them by advice, or to send a specialist to their assistance, but that where human life is concerned they have to take their chances and face illness and emergency in helpless ignorance."[31] Meigs believed that the ultimate success of the bureau's campaign to reduce high rates of maternal and infant mortality in rural populations depended upon health reformers' ability to solve two distinct but interrelated problems. First, good quality medical care remained inaccessible to a great many rural women. Poor roads, the lack of telephone service, and unreliable transportation constituted formidable obstacles standing between the provision of skilled medical services and the woman desperately in need of them. Further, the difficult conditions often encountered in rural areas served to drive up the cost of medical care. The long distances country physicians traveled in order to attend their patients meant that they could see relatively fewer of them and consequently they charged each patient a higher fee. "Where a prenatal visit, or a visit following labor means an additional $9.00 or $10.00, no unusual sum for a physician's visit in the country," Meigs explained, "it is naturally considered unattainable even by well-to-do country people." (Rural dwellers commonly balked at paying a physician's fees at all when he or she arrived too late to be present at the delivery.) Meigs's own proposal for reducing high rates of maternal and infant mortality in the country represented a sort of dual plan of attack in which early detection and hospital care would become more readily available for cases presenting obstetrical complications while access to skilled, in-home care would be increased to assist in more routine deliveries.[32]

But a second, more vexing, problem also underlay stubbornly high maternal and infant mortality rates in rural communities. Meigs believed that rural women themselves must be educated about the need for high quality medical care during pregnancy and labor. Country dwellers traditionally relied on self-help, especially the skills and experience of local women, to treat illnesses and accidents that were not life-threatening. Since the vast majority of childbirths resulted in healthy babies whose mothers survived, rural people tended not to view childbirth as an emergency requiring the expert services of a physician or professional midwife. The help of an experienced female relative or neighbor usually was deemed sufficient. When complications in childbirth did arise, however, the services of a skilled physician, nurse, or midwife often were not sought until it was too late, and many mothers and babies died tragically of causes that could have been prevented by a skilled caregiver.

The real problem, then, lay in ensuring that rural women received a diagnosis *before* the onset of labor that medical complications were likely to arise, a situation that required a trained health care provider. Many rural women simply did not see the need for the nonemergency services of health care professionals, as such routine health care duties fell within the purview of any competent farm wife. Meigs had faith that once rural women understood the efficacy of high quality medical care in reducing their own risks and those of their babies they would certainly insist on receiving it: "When women demand it, physicians will furnish it; medical colleges will provide better training for physicians; and communities, rural and urban, will see to it that women bearing children are properly protected."[33] Like the foreign-born mother in urban tenement neighborhoods, country mothers must be convinced that a higher standard of "good health" was attainable in an era of modern preventive health and hygiene practices. Toward this goal, Meigs made note of the crucial role filled by farm women's magazines as well as the bureau's own publications in disseminating the latest information on prenatal health care and the hygiene of pregnancy and infancy.

Local women's organizations represented another vital link between urban-based preventive health and hygiene campaigns and the rural residents of Illinois. Like their city sisters in Chicago, farm women joining campaigns to improve the health of country dwellers downstate adopted the language of maternalism in promoting their cause, utilizing their traditional role as the farm family's primary health care provider as a springboard for their participation in community activities. But the activities these women supported reflected their evolving middle-class identity as well, and prosperous farm women increasingly could be found supporting campaigns to clean up and beautify rural neighborhoods, purchasing commodities such as indoor plumbing to make the environments in their own homes more hygienic, and acquiring specialized domestic skills such as nutrition planning and healthful cooking to enhance the physical well-being of their families.

In 1918, the USDA undertook an inquiry into the various organizational activities being undertaken by rural women in America. Women's clubs, investigator Anne M. Evans asserted, "reduce the sense of drudgery inevitable to the woman who works alone every day. They bring women together for discussion of the problems of daily life in such a way that they may return to their work with a sense of companionship, renewed enthusiasm, and interest in their accomplishments." Like their urban counterparts, farm women's time would become free for participating in rural betterment activities such as improving public schools, increasing the enjoyment of family life, and crusading for maternal and child health reform. Evans was optimistic that such organized activities would result in "better home life on the farm, broader and bigger agricultural opportunities for the future, and an ideal rural community life." She illustrated her point with a description of the thriving Household Science Club of Wyanet, Illinois, where members delivered papers and listened to outside speakers on domestic science topics and planned various community improvement projects.[34] Ten years after President Theodore Roosevelt had appointed a special commission to address the problems of country life, Evans could report with satisfaction that Illinois farm women appeared to be doing their part in the rural rescue effort.

Rural women have a long history of organizational activity in the Midwest, and their formal and informal networks of support and service formed through communities, churches, schools and farming cooperatives had long constituted an important facet of farm life.[35] In the nineteenth century, many Illinois women became involved in agricultural reform movements such as the Farmers' Alliance and the Order of the Patrons of Husbandry, also known as the Grange. Grangers sought to improve their economic and social circumstances through cooperative ventures, education, and the promotion of progressive farming techniques. Women joined the Grange as full and equal members with men, rather than within segregated auxiliaries, a more customary way of organizing mixed-sex groups in the nineteenth century. Historian Donald B. Marti has argued that women's presence and participation lent an aura of "respectability" to Grange activities, and improving the status of women came to represent an inherent part of the vision of rural progress that Grangers developed; by 1893, the National Grange actively supported women's suffrage. The first Illinois Grange had been founded in 1868, and the number of new organizations in the state grew steadily, reaching more than 700 by 1875. Although its membership never grew to be exceedingly large, participation in the Grange had provided some rural women in Illinois with unprecedented opportunities to develop leadership and organizational skills as well as to exert political pressure for their own concerns. Women in the Illinois State Grange, for example, actively promoted a variety of causes including the establishment of kindergartens for early childhood education and the crusade against alcohol.[36]

A different type of rural reform organization also emerged in the middle of the nineteenth century. Farmers' Institutes became a popular means for agrarian men and women to meet for educational lectures, discussions, and entertainment. Sponsored by state-level departments of agriculture and by agricultural colleges, participation in the institutes topped 500,000 by 1900. In addition to papers on field-related topics presented by agricultural researchers and by farm men, the institutes also regularly featured presentations by women on farm production topics such as dairying, beekeeping, and poultry management — the traditional purview of the farm wife. By the end of the nineteenth century, however, the content of Farmers' Institutes programs for women reflected the growing influence of the new field of home economics with topics such as food preparation, home sanitation, and child care becoming more prominently featured.

In 1898, women in the Illinois Farmers' Institute founded a separate Department of Household Science within that organization.[37] Nora Mabel Dunlap, the "Mother of the Illinois Farmers' Institute," urged farm women in Illinois to take an active leadership role in improving the quality of rural life for themselves, their families, and their communities. Bettering the health of rural dwellers, especially of mothers and children, represented a crucial factor in advancing agricultural life, and topics pertaining to domestic hygiene and childhood nutrition as well as community sanitation consistently filled the agenda of the new women's department. The wife of a prominent state legislator, Dunlap's own commitment to the cause of rural health reform reportedly stemmed from the loss of all four of her children in infancy and early childhood. "She felt that if she had known more as a young mother about good nutrition, sanitation, and disease prevention," claimed a retrospective of her work in the Illinois Farmers' Institute, "some of the Dunlap children might have survived."[38]

Increasingly, programs presented at meetings of the Department of Household Science featured papers on various topics pertaining to rural public health, personal and family hygiene, and sanitary improvements for the home. Women meeting at the Illinois Farmers' Institute in 1919 were reminded of the seriousness of their responsibility for preventive health care: "If you take a preventable disease, it is your own fault," Caroline Geisel, a medical doctor as well as a "rousing personality" from Battle Creek, Michigan, admonished her audience. "Unless you are taking care of yourself, who is to finish your job when you leave this world untimely?" Enlightened farm women must act with diligence to ensure that their own health was not ruined, Geisel argued, for "You can't find a doctor to mend you once you are broken." In 1923, participants heard a lecture on rural sanitation by Dr. Thomas H. Leonard of the State Department of Public Health, complete with slides illustrating the proper and improper construction of water wells.[39] Rural club women's active interest in bettering the hygiene and sanitation of the farm home and community represented an assertion of both their traditional place as the rural family's primary medical practitioner and their right to perform that role using the latest, most advanced means available.

The University of Illinois, founded as a state agricultural college under the Morrill Land Grant Act of 1862, provided considerable support for the activities of rural women's clubs through its close association with the Illinois Farmers' Institute. In 1900, the university's school of home economics came under the zealous directorship of Isabel Bevier, a chemist and early leader in the home economics movement who had been a protegee of the field's chief founder, Ellen Richards, at the Massachusetts Institute of Technology. The newly revitalized school provided the women of the Farmers' Institute with speakers and demonstrations on various home economics topics. The overriding goal of women academics like Bevier was to establish the science of modern housekeeping as a serious intellectual pursuit at institutions of higher learning throughout the country. Ideally, female students trained in advanced scientific principles of household management at colleges and universities would then rigorously apply them in caring for their own homes and families. "Neither pious intentions nor fulsome oratory about the glories of motherhood furnish an adequate working basis for the serious study of the home," asserted Bevier. The discipline of home economics flourished in separate women's divisions of schools of agriculture at the nation's various land grant universities. During the winter months when farm chores became somewhat less arduous the University of Illinois offered "Schools for House-keepers" in which rural wives and mothers attended intensive short courses on farm home management. Programs promoting rural homemaking enjoyed a major boost in 1914 when Congress passed the Smith-Lever Act, which provided federal funds on a state-matching basis for agricultural education services. The act was intended to further the development of the extension work already being carried out by agricultural colleges as well as to extend those efforts more widely to rural counties throughout the United States. The USDA also expressed concern, however, about a perceived need for "more definite instruction in domestic and sanitary science and household art than is given to mixed audiences of the Farmers' Institutes."[40] The importance of farm women's role in advancing agrarian life, it seems, now required a higher degree of gender-specialized training than the Farmers' Institutes could offer. The new extension services funded by the Smith-Lever Act, therefore, would be more clearly segregated according to policymakers' ideas regarding appropriate gender activities for farm men and women.

In Illinois, Smith-Lever funds appropriated through the University of Illinois helped to sustain the county-based rural women's clubs known as "Home Bureaus." Club women themselves supplemented the federal funds through their membership fees, which ranged from $1.00 to $3.00 annually. The university provided extension agents known as "home advisors" who traveled to the county Home Bureau meetings giving lectures and demonstrations on various topics pertaining to farm household management. Home extension agents also trained local Home Bureau representatives to organize and carry out some of the demonstration work themselves. In using this particular organizational scheme, the USDA hoped to accomplish several things. First, this method allowed for the efficient dissemination of the latest research findings in domestic science to the largest numbers of rural wives and mothers. Second, extension administrators believed their mission would be more effectively fulfilled if the initiative and support for the Home Bureaus came from rural women themselves. Technically, extension agents were employees of both the university extension service *and* the members of the Home Bureaus, and the women of each local organization planned and carried out the work, elected officers, and handled their own bureau's funds. Third, this system was intended to stimulate interest in rural community welfare projects as well as to cultivate the leadership abilities of individual women. Finally, the organization of home extension services in Illinois was somewhat unique in that the Home Bureaus were established and maintained completely independently of the male-dominated, field-oriented Farm Bureaus.[41]

In the summer of 1915, the women of Kankakee County, Illinois, organized the first Home Bureau under the auspices of the Smith-Lever Act, raising $1,500 to employ Eva Benefiel as their local extension agent. Many years later Isabel Bevier recalled in her memoirs that the farm women of Kankakee County had approached her about establishing a separate women's organization, stating quite frankly that they found it impossible to work with the local Farm Bureau agent, believing "he was secretly working against them because he was jealous of their possible power." Four years later, seventeen county Home Bureaus with a combined membership of nearly 10,000 women had become active throughout the state. While technically the membership remained open to all women residing in the county, the Home Bureaus attracted proportionately more farm than nonfarm women. Home extension officials in Illinois attributed this interest on the part of farm women to the "greater complexity of the homemaking problems of the farm woman and her fewer opportunities for assistance." The farm women themselves, however, may have had more pragmatic reasons in mind. One woman, for example, said she enjoyed attending Home Bureau meetings because they gave her somewhere to meet with her neighbors besides funerals.[42]

The disparity between the high ideals of domestic science and the more immediate needs of farm women did, in fact, lead to periodic tensions, especially in the early years of the home extension service. As local-level missionaries of this new science, home extension agents were determined to raise their own status as educated professionals, and the type of instruction they offered often proved to be more theoretical than useful to the average farm woman, whose own work burdens and time constraints were already considerable. The profession of home extension agent was dominated by young, single, college-educated women. The "Illinois Plan" for training agents, for example, required that each candidate possess "a degree with major in home economics from a four year course in a university or recognized technical college . . . and a knowledge of life and maturity of judgment indicated by at least five years' experience in teaching or in lecturing and demonstrating or in actual farm life."[43] In addition to being well educated, home extension agents (often sporting bobbed hairstyles) raced around the countryside in automobiles and proficiently operated a variety of state-of-the art household technologies, an image that set them markedly apart from many of the women who were intended to be their clientele. Illinois home extension agent Clara Brian, for example, organized "equipment tours" in which she drove around McLean County, in the central region of the state, demonstrating vacuum cleaners, chemical toilets, gas mangles for ironing, and power washing machines in farm homes. Brian reportedly logged a total of 3,354 automobile miles in 1919. The farm women in Brian's audience may well have been amazed by Brian's newfangled technologies; but the extent to which they could have incorporated them into their own work routines is unclear, for less than 10 percent of Illinois farm homes were wired for electricity at this time.[44]

During the early years of Isabel Bevier's tenure at the University of Illinois, women in the Illinois Farmers' Institute were so distrustful of her emphasis on abstract theoretical science and experimental methods that they nearly forced her resignation from the university. They did succeed in closing down the university's fully electrified and equipped demonstration home (complete with the latest in furnishings brought down from Chicago), which they viewed as irrelevant to the work they actually did on the farm. "What women of the rural districts seem to want," representatives of the Farmers' Institute explained to Dean Davenport of the university's College of Agriculture, "is training along practical lines to fit them for housekeepers of moderate means rather than [as] teachers of the higher branches." Bevier, in turn, expressed a certain amount of contempt toward the women of the Illinois Farmers' Institute, whose own efforts on behalf of farm women's advancement she once described as being "haphazard" and "well-intentioned but uneducational."[45]

The new Home Bureaus targeted a more progressive, educated, and prosperous group of farm women than the predominant membership of the older Illinois Farmers' Institute. The programs carried out by the USDA's extension services strongly promoted the image of the modernized farm home as a means to advance agrarian life, an image that highlighted the farm woman's increasing function as a consumer rather than a producer of goods and services. This shift in perceptions about farm women's appropriate gender role is well illustrated by historian Joan M. Jensen's observation that the houses of wealthier farm families in this period began to have smaller kitchens, separate dining rooms, and larger parlors; in other words, the farm home was increasingly arranged around an ideal of female domesticity rather than of farm women's productivity.[46] The urban middle-class ideal of domesticity that informed a large portion of the content of home extension activities is clearly reflected in the credo composed for the Illinois

Home Bureaus by Juliet Lita Bane, who directed home economics extension work at the University of Illinois from 1918 to 1923. The credo was widely reprinted in home extension service publications:

The Aim of the Home Bureau

The ideal sought is to have every home —
Economically sound
Mechanically convenient
Physically healthful
Morally wholesome
Artistically satisfying
Mentally stimulating
Socially responsible
Spiritually inspiring
Founded upon mutual affection
     and respect

Home Bureau programs promoting rural health reform rested on the assumption that all rural women, once they were properly instructed in the fundamentals of preventive health care and household hygiene, stood ready and able to take whatever steps were necessary to elevate their own health standards as well as those of their communities. But the attainment of better rural health represented an important piece of the larger modernization message promoted by the home extension service, and thus health reform campaigns were closely tied to the acquisition of household technologies which would help transform farm families and households into closer approximations of their urban, middle-class counterparts. When Juliet Lita Bane delivered a series of talks on the subject of children's health, for example, her lectures covered a range of topics including nutrition, proper clothing, personal hygiene, home sanitation, lighting, heating, and even household budgeting. Clara Brian's preventive health care presentations at McLean County Home Bureau meetings featured magic lantern slides of sanitary and unsanitary toilet facilities followed by pictures of healthy children to remind her audiences just why indoor plumbing constituted a basic necessity for the modern farm family. Centered around the acquisition of consumer products, the ideal of modern, urban, middle-class domesticity that home extension programs projected remained beyond the reach of many farm families in Illinois.[47]

Further, the USDA's faith that new technologies would release farm women for crucial "uplift" activities such as health reform in rural communities failed to address the fact that not all rural dwellers enjoyed equal access to the modern conveniences that would make such a transition possible. To begin with, while farm households may have been acquiring modern technologies such as automobiles and farm machinery, it is less clear to what extent women actually controlled their use. Secondly, as historians of women's household labor have pointed out, the proliferation of various "labor-saving" devices for the home have not necessarily reduced the amount of work performed by women, they have only changed the nature of that work.[48] Finally, the emerging cadre of modern mothers who did gain enough leisure time to join rural women's clubs represented only the relatively small group of farm families who prospered in this era.

At the same time farm mothers were being encouraged to form networks for social activism within their local communities, those communities were themselves becoming economically stratified. In Illinois, the geographical distribution of the newly forming Home Bureaus is revealing, for they appeared disproportionately in that state's wealthier northern and central regions. Five years after their initiation in Kankakee County, for example, fifteen Home Bureaus operated in the northern two-thirds of the state while only two clubs had been organized in the southern third. A 1928 study of home extension services in Vermilion County, in the central portion of the state, found that participants were more likely to be from larger, wealthier, family owned farms. Conversely, this study found that tenant farmers and women from the county's smaller farms participated much less frequently in home extension activities.[49]

Campaigns promoting rural health reform in Illinois nurtured the development of the modern rural mother who would take her place alongside her urban, middle-class counterpart in health and social welfare activism. While the lofty plans of reformers and the more prosaic needs of farm women occasionally resulted in conflict, it is important to keep in mind that a large measure of initiative came from rural women themselves. Home Bureau members, for example, planned and organized their own meetings, selected program topics, and invited guest speakers; Home Bureau advisors' salaries were always at least partially supported by membership fees. Middle-class club women in rural areas and small towns often initiated their own projects designed to improve community health standards. In 1919, for example, members of the Williamson County Home Bureau enlisted the aid of public health officers and children from public and parochial schools in exterminating the "breeding places of flies." The women then extended their campaign by delivering addresses on "the necessity of having a clean town" to audiences at moving picture shows; they even spoke to local meetings of the miners' union. When in 1926 three cases of typhoid fever were reported in Champaign County, women of the local Home Bureau supervised a survey of the water quality of all wells used by local school children. The same year, Champaign County Home Bureau members announced their own plans for a "positive health campaign," urging local physicians, dentists, and nurses to assist them in "making wives capable of cooperating with doctors" by training them in home nursing procedures.[50]

This kind of female initiative was actively encouraged by the home extension service. Isabel Bevier claimed that, upon her arrival at the University of Illinois, she found local women to be "handicapped in their efforts for leadership" within the Farmers' Institute. "Most of the plans were made and executed by the men," Bevier recalled. "In those days, women were very timid, afraid of the sound of their own voice in a public audience." The gender-segregated Home Bureaus had been explicitly designed to correct this perceived imbalance of power and to encourage women in rural areas to assert their rightful place as guardians of family and community health. The University of Illinois's Fannie Brooks tried to encourage the development of local women's leadership skills, for example, by traveling throughout the state conducting training schools at which Home Bureau members learned how to present preventive health care demonstrations in their own communities.[51]

Preventive health and hygiene campaigns in downstate Illinois granted a special status to women—especially to farm mothers—as the guardians of health and well-being for rural families and communities. A long history of independence and isolation meant that farm women were by tradition the primary health care practitioners for their families, and health reformers sought to enhance and to modernize this role. Through local club activities many rural wives and mothers received vital information on effective home sanitation methods and learned valuable lessons in maternal and infant hygiene. For many women, monitoring sanitary conditions in the rural community became an extension of their traditional role in health care provision. Evidence from farm periodicals and USDA surveys in the period from approximately 1910 to 1930 indicates that a particular segment of midwestern farm women—generally native-born and middle-class—began to interpret poor rural health conditions as evidence of their *own* oppression as well. In the movement toward healthier communities and more hygienic homes in Illinois, these "wide-awake" farm mothers were not about to be left behind.

At the same time, however, the emerging preeminence of the USDA's home extension services as a means of mobilizing rural women meant that the orientation of health reform programs would become increasingly privatized and consumer-oriented, an integral part of the broader modernization message the service continued to promote throughout the 1920s. Although downstate women took a great deal of interest in health reform campaigns, the considerable expense involved in acquiring modern conveniences such as indoor plumbing kept some of the most basic means of health improvement beyond the reach of many of them. As modernizing farm mothers took up the banner of health reform from their sisters in Chicago, agricultural life itself was becoming increasingly stratified by class.

4

Exhibiting Health

In 1915, an exhibit in the Illinois State Armory building at Springfield displayed the findings of an extensive survey of living and working conditions conducted in the capital city the previous year. The survey's sponsor, the Russell Sage Foundation, explained that the exhibit had been designed expressly to "present the major findings in such simple, graphic, and entertaining ways as to gain the attention and be understood by the many, particularly those who are not habitual readers of periodicals or printed reports." Planned, constructed, and operated largely by Springfield citizens themselves, the exhibit reportedly attracted several thousand visitors during its ten-day run. The exhibitors devoted five separate sections to portraying problematic public health conditions in Springfield and promoting their improvement through cooperative efforts in both the public and private spheres. Several maps, for example, demonstrated chronic health hazards stemming from impure local water supplies by delineating how polluted water from the Sangamon River flowed into the homes of Springfield families.[1]

Conditions affecting infants and children received a special emphasis at the Russell Sage exhibit. One panel promoting the need for more accurate collection of birth registration data featured a colorful banner pleading "Count Your Family, Father Springfield." The most dramatic presentation of all, however, depicted the surprisingly high infant mortality rates the Sage survey had uncovered in this midsized midwestern city. Entitled "The Tenth Baby," the display featured watercolor portraits of ten "winsome baby faces" grouped together on a panel. The last face, painted on ground glass, pulsated as an electric light flashed through the glass, calling attention to "the tenth baby that does not reach its first birthday" in Springfield. Bold lettering on the poster admonished curious onlookers that "the city could save most of these babies by employing public health nurses to instruct the mothers." The subject of children's health was also dramatized in several plays presented during exhibition hours, written and performed by local residents. One play portrayed school children being attacked by imp characters representing childhood diseases. The imps, revelling in their success in making children sick, performed a "mad dance" until a team of doctors and nurses arrived on the scene and carted them off in a patrol wagon.[2]

The crowds of spectators visiting the Springfield exhibit that year added their numbers to the thousands who participated in a vigorous and varied statewide movement to bring the message of modernization through better health directly to the people of Illinois. Entertaining, frequently whimsical, and often highly dramatic, these spectacles imparted the latest scientific information on subjects such as personal hygiene, nutrition, normal childhood growth and development, and household and community sanitation in an effort to render them more accessible to the lay public. Newly available technologies such as electrical lighting and motion picture projection systems allowed these exhibits to convey modernity through the medium as well as the substance of the display. Although they had been wary of "cheap amusements" initially, Illinois health reformers eventually learned to make their own uses of the mass media and commercialized leisure activities that were becoming an ever-larger part of the midwestern cultural landscape in this era.[3]

Integrally tied to broader themes of Americanizing immigrants in Chicago's tenement blocks and uplifting rural residents of the state, health reformers carried preventive health and hygiene campaigns to agricultural fairs, grade school pageants, movie houses, and church socials throughout Illinois. Summer Chautauqua programs, for example, featured sessions with titles such as "What is Health?" and "Fever Nursing" as standard offerings. For their extensive efforts, Illinois health reformers were rewarded with large and enthusiastic audiences as both urban and rural dwellers admired infant competitors at better baby contests, watched demonstrations on the proper care and feeding of children, and listened attentively to public lectures on a range of medical topics presented by health care professionals.[4]

Illinois health reformers designed many of their campaigns to popularize preventive health and hygiene expressly for a female audience. With an eye toward reaching as many mothers in the state as possible, the Illinois State Board of Health began distributing the first of its circulars on the subject of infant care in 1905. *Infant Feeding* emphasized hygienic feeding practices, offered advice concerning the baby's diet, weaning, and artificial feeding, stressed the potential hazards of patent medicines, and provided prescriptions for the general care of the infant, especially during the hot summer months when hundreds of Illinois children perished from "summer complaint," or dehydration following a severe bout with diarrhea. The special virtue of the circular, according to its publishers, was that it was written "not for physicians, but for mothers," and that authors had taken care so that the topics presented were "dwelt upon so clearly and so concisely that any woman of average intelligence may read and understand." In addition to newborn care, the circular included advice to the new mother on her own health during the postpartum period as well. The pamphlet proved to be quite popular, especially with rural and small-town mothers in Illinois whose access to prenatal medical services remained severely limited, and the State Board of Health quickly distributed several thousand copies. Regional newspapers such as the *St. Louis Republic* praised the pamphlet for its clear, direct writing style, avoidance of technical medical terms, and use of easy-to-follow illustrations.[5] The pamphlet's wide acceptance among Illinois mothers prompted the publication of a new edition in 1909. Now entitled *The Care of the Baby*, the circular had grown to thirty-two pages and included lavish illustrations featuring attractive and apparently well-fed babies.

When the booklet underwent yet another major revision in 1916, the publication of *Our Babies: How to Keep Them Well and Happy* was praised by Governor Dunne as a "service to the commonwealth and especially to our baby citizens." The governor also revealed that Mrs. Dunne, herself the mother of thirteen children, somehow had found the time to read the new publication and had been very impressed as well. But motherhood itself was changing, and by 1916 a number of problems distinctive to modern child rearing had to be addressed. In addition to the customary warnings concerning the use of patent medicines, unsanitary bottle feeding, and too little fresh air that had served as staple lessons in the earlier versions, the new edition advised mothers against taking their babies to moving picture shows and other popular entertainments where their little ones' sensitive nervous systems might become overstimulated. Supported by a steady demand from Illinois mothers, the state public health agency's roster of publications concerning children's health topics grew steadily, and by 1923 the list featured a number of new titles including "Prenatal Care and Baby's Health," "Infantile Paralysis," and "How to Fight the Fly."[6]

Volunteer support provided by women's organizations was critical to the success of popular health reform activities in both urban and rural areas of the state. Although a 1901 statute had mandated the formation of boards of health for all territories located outside of incorporated cities and villages in Illinois, a dearth of funding and negligible political support had impaired the development of public health efforts for decades. The state had been divided into 1,100 separate public health districts, the vast majority of which were too small to be sustained by local taxes. While the slogan "public health is purchasable" remained a perennial favorite among public health advocates in this period, at least one Illinois health commissioner noted that "in the small towns and villages the price may be so high as to be almost prohibitive." Further, public health officials were politically appointed in Illinois, and as late as 1919 only 169 individuals serving as district health officers had received any medical training. The extremely decentralized structure of public health services outside of Chicago left open plenty of space in which grassroots women's activism on behalf of improving the public's health could flourish. The efforts of rural women's organizations in supporting health campaigns in downstate Illinois mirrored those of middle-class and elite women's associations in Chicago. The Children's Bureau, in conjunction with the National Federation of Women's Clubs, had designated one week in March as National Baby Week and urged active participation in this campaign by women's organizations throughout the country. Illinois women responded to the call.[7]

The Woman's Club of Flora, a southern Illinois town with a population of a little over 2,700, organized an entire week of activities promoting the improvement of children's health in their community. After corresponding with both the Illinois State Board of Health and the Children's Bureau, the women of Flora had secured pamphlets, moving picture shows, magic lantern slides, and exhibits for a mass meeting to be held at the local opera house. "A program is being prepared," club members promised readers of the *Southern Illinois Record*, "that will interest and instruct everyone and of course, is free to all." Hoping to fill in existing gaps within the public health infrastructure of the state, health reformers from both the Children's Bureau and the Illinois State Board of Health actively encouraged this kind of local, female-led initiative.[8]

Among the most prominent downstate organizations promoting popular health reform efforts in this era were the county-based Home Bureaus that linked local rural women's activities to the extension services of the U.S. Department of Agriculture. Home extension had been instituted in order to facilitate the farm woman's entrance into civic life by both diminishing her daunting workload on the family farm and extending her ability to reach out into the local community to form networks with other activist women.[9] The farm mother's traditional responsibility as her family's primary health care practitioner meant that topics concerning health regularly occupied a position of central importance within extension programs. Subjects such as home care of the sick, emergency first aid, and household sanitary measures became steady fare at local Home Bureau meetings. Traveling exhibits known as "movable schools" brought preventive health and hygiene education to small towns and rural villages throughout the state. From 1915 to 1916, for example, a movable school featuring the subject "nursing and health" traveled to twenty-six counties in Illinois. Home demonstration agents gave 168 lectures on health care in conjunction with the exhibit, which made its appearance at high schools, women's club meetings, Sunday schools, and the Illinois Chautauqua. Over 32,000 people reportedly attended movable school events during the period from September 1916 to September 1917.[10] In 1915 the University of Illinois hired public health nurse Fannie Brooks to supervise all of the preventive health education activities being conducted under the auspices of the home extension service. Brooks developed an ambitious — and for busy farm women, an exceedingly demanding — "positive health program" within which she intended "to stimulate self-study to attain health individually, to improve household sanitation including the disposal of sewerage and the improvement of the water supply, to arouse interest in community health, and to obtain community sanitary conditions tending to promote health." A special aim of Brooks's positive health program was to provide expectant mothers in rural Illinois with information "regarding their general care during pregnancy, labor, and the convalescing period and to reduce mortality among mothers and infants." Brooks cooperated with the Illinois State Board of Health in conducting maternal and infant health lectures, supervising the weighing and measuring of babies at mobile well-baby clinics, and setting up child welfare displays at Home Bureau meetings. She designed a series of lessons especially "for the expectant mother and for the mother of a babe under nine months of age" among members of the local Champaign County Home Bureau. In discussing preventive health care, Brooks urged her female audiences to avoid relying on patent medicines, a persistent rural custom which Illinois health reformers found particularly vexing. Hoping to encourage a more enlightened approach to preventive health, Brooks devised a chart on which individuals could keep track of their health habits, including the number of hours they slept, the glasses of water they drank, and the amount of exercise they received each day. "If you follow this daily health program," she instructed them, "you will realize that patent medicines are unnecessary."[11]

The extension service's health education programs proved to be extremely popular among rural Illinois women; activities featuring children's health care found an especially receptive audience in downstate communities. In the period from 1917 to 1918, for example, 4,431 women throughout the state attended home extension lectures on child health and infant feeding. One farm woman declared that "if the Home Bureau were nothing more than a child care and training class, it would be worth all it cost." Clara Brian, McLean County's Home Bureau advisor, related the story of one woman who, having followed the extension service's advice on infant feeding, referred to her child as "our Home Bureau baby, because she is so healthy and well." The women of the Champaign County Home Bureau even took partial credit for a perfect score received at a baby contest held at the state fair. Baby Graycroft's success was largely due, they asserted, to the fact that his mother "secured help from the extension service on prenatal feeding, and afterwards followed out the Home Bureau program in nutrition and child feeding supplemented by conferences with the home advisor."[12]

Under its third director, C. St. Clair Drake, the Illinois State Board of Health also began to put more concerted effort into popularizing public health education, broadcasting its preventive health and hygiene messages as widely as possible throughout the state. Drake, a Canadian who had graduated from the Chicago Homeopathy Medical College in 1891, headed the agency from 1914 to 1921. Drake refashioned the rather dry monthly compilation of statistical reports which had served as the Board's official organ into the *Illinois Health News*, a considerably more approachable publication— complete with lively cover illustrations and sprinkled throughout with cartoons, quips, and humorous anecdotes—through which Drake intended to "reduce the technical science of preventive medicine in terms of practical application for the individual and the community." Seeking "a new and larger audience," *Illinois Health News* provided up-to-date information on disease and death rates in the state and gave coverage to local epidemics and other public health emergencies such as floods and tornadoes. Extensive publicity was also given to local health reform projects undertaken by women's clubs. The inaugural issue in January 1915 announced that the new publication was meant to be "merely a part of a definite campaign of popular public health education contemplated by the State Board of Health."[13]

During the first decades after its inception in 1877, the board's activities had been largely limited to licensing medical practitioners, but by the mid-1910s the functions of this statewide public health agency had changed dramatically. In July 1917, Drake presided over a major structural reorganization in which the responsibility for registering health care professionals was split off into a separate department and the board itself reconstituted as the State

Department of Public Health, an essentially new agency intending to focus more directly on matters of sanitation, education, and disease control "freed of all embarrassing burdens" associated with enforcing the Medical Practice Act. The reorganization scheme, which had been prompted by a strong recommendation from the U.S. Public Health Service, included the establishment of a special Division of Child Hygiene and Public Health Nursing to carry out much of the educational effort.[14]

Under Drake's administration the statewide health agency introduced a series of innovations such as the wildly popular better baby contests featured at the annual Illinois State Fair and special theme weeks highlighting the work of local health and social welfare organizations. Traveling exhibits on topics ranging from prenatal care to the prevention of tuberculosis were made available by the department for use by community clubs and local health and social welfare agencies in their own activities. Several exhibits were designed specifically for the edification of children, and displays with titles such as "The A-1 American Girl," "The A-1 American Boy," and "Babes in Healthland" traveled to schools, churches, recreation centers, and youth gatherings sponsored by 4-H and the Girl Scouts. Local fairs, Farmers' Institutes, and the meetings of community organizations and women's clubs frequently served as venues for exhibits promoting preventive health and hygiene education. Various medical and nonmedical professionals, including Red Cross nurses, public health workers, and agricultural extension agents, gave lectures and led question-and-answer sessions in conjunction with the exhibits. While local audiences regularly flocked to presentations on health topics, colorful stereopticon slide shows with titles such as "What Every Baby Wants" and "Give the Baby a Fair Deal" could be added to these local programs in order to attract even greater crowds.[15]

Public health officials soon discovered that exhibits utilizing mechanized models represented an especially effective way to draw in curious crowds and relay to them important information about preventive health and hygiene. By the mid-1910s the State Board of Health had developed several models complete with such attention-grabbing features as flashing electric lights and moving figurines. These novel exhibits could be borrowed by community groups for display at local functions — provided that they could secure an experienced operator to handle the electrical equipment. One especially elaborate presentation at the 1914 Illinois State Fair even garnered publicity in the national media including the influential social reform journal, *The Survey*, which took special note of the exhibit's "originality, importance and general attractiveness."

One of the several displays in this extensive exhibit featured, among other things, a mechanical model that depicted the health dangers posed by polluted water from shallow wells, a hazard that remained all too common in a great many rural Illinois communities. While two dolls appeared to be drawing water from an outdoor pump, water leaking from a nearby privy vault and barn could be seen draining into the well that supplied the pump. A sign above the model warned: "Shallow dug wells dig many deep graves." Another display, intended to portray "an honest illustration of just what the open window will do to the air of the sleeping room" contrasted conditions in two bedrooms, one with windows open and the other with windows closed. A doll occupied a bed in each room. Smoke pumped out through the dolls' nostrils by means of a mechanical device operated by an electric motor quickly clouded the chamber with the closed windows while the other room remained blissfully clear. A third model dramatized "The Dirty Fly in Action." Mechanical flies buzzed back and forth from a barn and pig sty to a house where a doll family was seated to dinner at the kitchen table. Another doll lay sick in an upstairs bedroom, presumably expiring of typhoid fever. Telling the "fly story more graphically than words or pictures can ever do," the State Board of Health noted that the latter display seemed to be a particular favorite with the crowd. Over sixty feet long and weighing over 3,600 pounds, this intricately designed health exhibit traveled from Springfield at the close of the state fair to be featured at industrial shows, medical society meetings, schools, and women's club functions throughout the state.[16]

Buoyed by the success of the 1914 exhibit, the State Board of Health developed a number of additional new displays, including several that focused on children's health topics specifically. Many of these seemed to have been designed for maximum shock effect, making preventive health and hygiene lessons even more memorable to the audiences viewing them. A seven-foot-long, 475-pound electrical model, for example, presented a smallpox epidemic in the form of an erupting volcano. Smoke bellowed out from the crater until the smallpox vaccination, symbolized by an electrically lighted candlesnuffer, was lowered onto the volcano thereby cutting off the eruption. One particularly macabre spectacle featured a mechanical model in the foreground which consisted of baby dolls attached to a revolving cylinder. Above each cylinder crouched "a skeleton figure of death that cuts down with his sickle every tenth and twentieth doll respectively." In the background, a painted scene depicting a forlorn cemetery showed "the eternal resting place of the innocent victims." Entitled "Infant Death Rate," this exhibit undoubtedly drew considerable attention at any community function in which it might have appeared.[17]

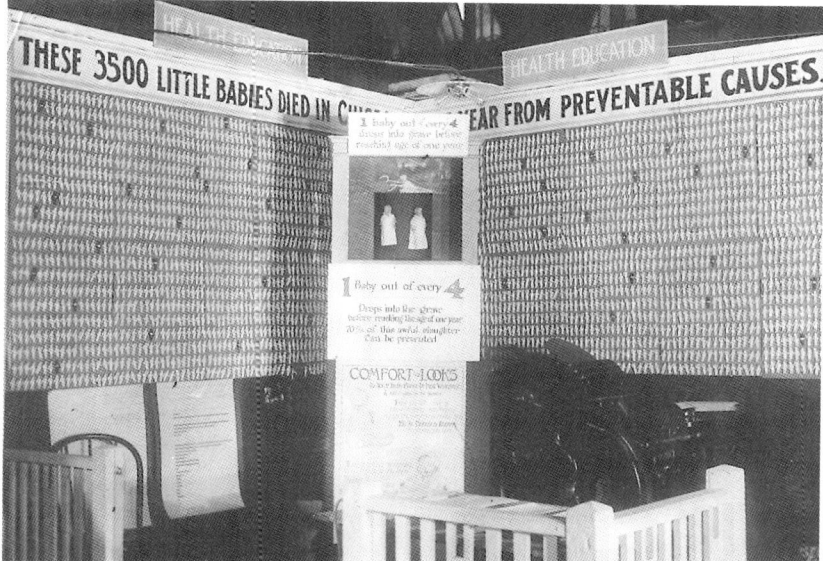

Figure 4.1. Illinois State Board of Health child welfare exhibit, Chicago, Illinois, 1911 (photographer unknown). Chicago Historical Society, photograph ICHi-26727.

Motion pictures also began to find their way into public health exhibits. Early in the century, during the heyday of the cheap urban nickelodeon, reformers had been leery of the potential of movies to do harm to the physical and social well-being of the American public. Activists in large industrial cities had noted with some trepidation the powerful draw that silent pictures seemed to have for immigrant audiences, including foreign-born mothers and their daughters. As historians Stuart Ewen and Elizabeth Ewen have noted, silent movies projected images of American culture in a language of image, sign, and gesture that immigrant audiences often found more comprehensible than the language spoken by native residents, rendering these early films into significant agents of acculturation. But the mass appeal of moving images quickly reached beyond the urban areas where they had first been introduced, and by 1910 movie houses had become permanent fixtures in small towns as well as in large cities. Motion pictures carried indelible images of urban consumer culture to rural audiences, who eagerly absorbed the underlying modernization messages these films conveyed along with adventure stories and melodrama.[18]

In 1914 the Russell Sage Foundation survey looked into the movie-going habits of the residents of Springfield, Illinois, who by this time could choose from among ten different permanent movie theaters in their city with a total seating capacity of 3,232. While the investigators found that the theater facilities themselves were generally clean and well-ventilated (deeming only two to be in less than satisfactory condition) and the character of the entertainments themselves of "average wholesomeness," they did express concern that the city provided "no machinery for regular inspection" in order to monitor "moral and sanitary conditions" in its movie houses. "What assurance is there that objectionable features will not surreptitiously creep into them?" the investigators asked in alarm. "Should it not be somebody's job to see that they are kept out?" Toward that end, the survey's final report included a model ordinance for licensing and regulating motion picture houses that it recommended civic leaders adopt in their home towns. Perhaps of most concern to the Sage Foundation investigators, however, was the amount of time that Springfield's youth apparently spent at the movies. Self-reporting among both boys and girls of high-school age revealed that the total number of attendances at motion picture shows was three times that for any other form of leisure-time entertainment including dances, parties, and plays. (Investigators compared the Springfield figures to similar data collected for youth in several cities in Iowa, pointing out that "the movie habit is stronger in Springfield than it is in Iowa.") Such concerns were not limited to the downstate region, however, and civic reformers also monitored the movie-going habits of Chicago's youth. In 1917, for example, the Woman's City Club instituted a special subcommittee to investigate the issue of "better films for children," hoping eventually to replace the questionable fare currently being offered to young audiences in their city.[19]

Other prominent Progressive Era reformers, however, realized that motion pictures held enormous potential for instructing and edifying the masses and, carefully handled, could serve as a social benefit rather than a public menace. Contributing to the construction of a new genre that historian Kay Sloan has called the "social problem film," some progressive reformers even made movies themselves. In 1913 Jane Addams, for instance, starred in a film promoting women's suffrage while a melodrama made by Margaret Sanger addressed the issue of civil liberties. Illinois health reformers caught on to movies' potential rather quickly, and by the mid-1910s motion pictures could be viewed alongside the posters and mechanical models being displayed at public health exhibits. In 1915, for example, the Woman's City Club urged its members to attend a "worthy exhibit" on the subject of health being held at the Civic Club of Chicago that featured a film presentation as part of the evening program. The following year the *Illinois Health News* even spoofed health and social welfare reformers' newfound propensity for utilizing the modern medium of motion pictures by presenting a series of cartoon sketches on the subject of birth registration that had been drawn to mimic movie stills. "These days," the caption read, "every social movement has a movie all its own."[20]

But of all the preventive health movement's innovations in extending the modernization message to the masses, none proved to be more popular than the better baby contest. Historian Alisa Klaus has traced the origins of this "uniquely American" approach to children's health care to two Iowa club women working independently of the male professional medical establishment. Endorsed by the Children's Bureau, baby contests became a standard feature at rural women's club meetings, public health demonstrations, and, most significantly, at state and local agricultural fairs. Local newspapers and the farm press facilitated the rapid dissemination of the baby contest idea throughout the Midwest; some magazines even sponsored contests of their own. In Illinois, public health officials believed that contests held in conjunction with agricultural fairs with their "great crowds of people . . . from town and country and the great interest in 'prize winners' of all kinds," would provide an invaluable means for publicizing children's health care throughout the state. Further, they believed they could better promote principles of proper hygiene among rural mothers by modeling a sanitary nursery environment while judges — sometimes costumed in surgical gowns — stressed the importance of seeking regular checkups from a family physician.[21]

Thus, this popular children's health reform activity also carried the important function of socializing rural mothers into their new, modern role as conscientious consumers of domestic hygiene goods and health care services. "Here is an unusual opportunity to secure a thorough examination of your baby free of charge," urged Mrs. William Downey of the Illinois Farmers' Institute in announcing the addition of a baby contest to the program of the Institute's annual meeting in 1916. "If you have a 100 per cent baby, Illinois ought to know about it. If your baby has defects which cause him to be scored low, you ought to know about it." The first statewide better baby contest was held in the Women's Building at the 1915 Illinois State Fair in Springfield, where, aided by members of the "ladies auxiliary," 250 child participants were examined by contest personnel.[22]

Baby contests reflected the emerging field of pediatric medicine's preoccupation with establishing normative standards of child development as the young contestants were weighed, measured, and given a series of physical and "mental" tests for which they were awarded points in various categories.

The State Department of Public Health stressed that baby contest judges should consist only of "specially trained experts" and devised a standardized scorecard based on a model issued by the American Medical Association. The board's guidelines required judges to scrutinize the child's head, scalp, chest, abdomen, arms and hands, genitalia, legs and feet, posture and gait, nose, mouth, teeth, throat, and skin. Normative standards for children's mental development were also evolving in this period, and these became a standard part of the baby contest examination as well. By the age of six months, for example, babies were expected to be able to sit up without support, hold their heads steadily, and turn to look in the direction of unexpected noises. At twelve months, a baby should stand unsupported, repeat a few syllables, and imitate the examiners' movements. Other "mental tests" administered in the contests rated the baby's level of attentiveness, facial expression, and apparent overall disposition.[23]

The state health department provided contest organizers with rather detailed descriptions of what characteristics should be deemed a "defect" in each category, as well as the number of points to be deducted from the contestant's score. Evidence of rickets, for example, was to be penalized, as was any curvature of the spine, asymmetry of the limbs, scaling or diseased skin or scalp, or excessive deviations from an established standard in the child's height or weight. In providing specifications in such exacting — if not always medically significant — detail, public health officials hoped to elevate the contests into something beyond mere baby beauty pageants. Rather, these "conferences" were to be treated as "modern" and "scientific" events with important educational and health benefits for parents, children, and the rural community at large. Interestingly, in some cases the baby contests' rigorously prescribed procedures for children's health examinations actually exceeded the professional training of local physicians. The medical doctor scrutinizing children at the 1916 Illinois Farmers' Institute contest, for example, was forced to confess that "this is a new proposition to we physicians as well as to you mothers. Most of us have never had the experience of examining children for such tests as this."[24]

A particular advantage of holding baby contests at agricultural fairs was the potential to reach a great many farm mothers who, because of their geographic isolation, economic circumstances, or lack of time away from chores might not otherwise have been able to see that their children received thorough health examinations. But just as important, health reformers believed, was the need to socialize rural mothers to seek professional medical advice for their family's preventive health maintenance rather than following the rural tradition of calling on doctors in cases of dire emergency only. Although the examiners themselves were not exclusively medical doctors — contest organizers commonly recruited nurses, social workers, and kindergarten teachers for the job — public health officials believed that better baby contests would prove to be invaluable to farm mothers for the advice and assistance regarding their children's health care they gained by participating. Contest organizers made it a point to stress to rural mothers the importance of following up their children's examinations with regular visits to a qualified medical doctor.

Public health officials repeatedly emphasized the serious educational purposes underlying the irresistible entertainment value of babies on display. One crucial means for conveying this seriousness of purpose was the maintenance of strict hygiene measures at the contest site itself. The state health department stood adamant in asserting that baby contests should bring home the lesson of "absolute cleanliness" to all participants — as well as to the legions of observers who jammed the exhibition halls in order to catch a glimpse of the proceedings. Soap, water, and paper towels were to be much in evidence throughout the examinations, public health officials directed, and judges must clearly be seen washing their hands before and after handling each baby. The examining rooms themselves were designed to mimic the setting of a modern sanitary hospital or clinic as well as to serve as a model of proper household hygiene in the rural or urban modern home. Contest guidelines directed that any woodwork should be "painted white with a high gloss finish" and the floors preferably would be covered in white or light-colored linoleum. All persons coming in contact with child contestants were required to wear surgical gowns over their street clothes. "A soiled apron or neglected finger nails on the part of a nurse or examiner," public health officials admonished, "may undo the benefits of a thousand wise sayings and a score of high-sounding lectures."[25]

While contest organizers firmly believed in the intrinsic value of a free, up-to-date health examination, they offered the further enticement of prizes to mothers whose babies achieved the highest scores. Many health reformers considered cash prizes to be vulgar and feared that offering money would provide an inappropriate incentive for mothers' participation. Nevertheless, local contest organizers did sometimes offer cash awards as well as plaques and trophies. Prizewinners at the Illinois State Fair received savings bank deposits and, in the contest's early years, the recipients of the prestigious Mother's Award for highest-scoring child in any category received a "lady's gold watch, valued at one hundred and twenty-five dollars." It soon became clear, however, that such pecuniary incentives to mothers for bringing in their children for health examinations conflicted with the economic interests of local physicians in private practice who provided crucial scientific prestige as well as much-needed volunteer manpower to the contests. Within a few years, the lady's gold watch was replaced by a silver cup.[26]

Photographs of prizewinning children were often published in local newspapers and farm journals; in 1919, for example, a party of midwestern state governors and former governors posed for photographers, "each Governor holding in his arms a smiling Illinois baby." *Illinois Health News* occasionally featured contest winners on its front cover. Indeed, photographing the winning child represented an important element in baby contests specifically designed to attract the participation of rural mothers, and the baby's photograph itself was sometimes bestowed as a prize. A contest sponsored by the Springfield magazine *The Farm Home*, for example, offered a formal baby portrait to the mother of the first-place winner. Mothers in small towns and rural areas highly valued photographs of their children, especially formal portraits, as both an emblem of their family's heritage and a symbol of their own attainment of the special status of motherhood.[27]

Prizes such as cash and formal baby portraits served as a powerful inducement to rural mothers' participation, but what were the consequences for those whose babies did not compete successfully in these events? Contest promoters argued that it was precisely these children and their mothers for whom the event would prove to be most valuable in the long run. Illinois public health officials invited the mothers of babies who received low scores at the state fair to attend informal sessions in which they would be advised by "a staff of consultants" on how to improve their children's health. In this way, mothers in rural areas and small towns would be assured of receiving the latest information about what was considered to be a "sound" or "normal" baby — and why their own children may have fallen short of the mark. To further emphasize the long-term benefits of participation, contest organizers at the Illinois State Fair created a special category for judging children showing the greatest degree of improvement from the previous year's event.[28]

Indeed, some child welfare activists appeared extremely uncomfortable with the inherently competitive nature of the better baby contest — and, perhaps, with the display of ambition on the part of many aspiring mothers who entered their children as well. Although in their publications Illinois public health officials consistently used the less competitive-sounding term "baby conference," as suggested by the federal Children's Bureau, state fair organizers within the Illinois Department of Agriculture continued to refer to them as "contests" in their own records and dutifully recorded entrants and winners alongside those participating in livestock competitions. Health reformers hoped to soften the competitive spirit by including a special division in which children could receive health examinations without being entered for competition. Further, public health officials stressed that, in theory at least, any mother, regardless of her economic or social standing, could enter her child into a baby contest — and any mother's child could be pronounced the winner. "As in all other features of public health work," they asserted, "rich and poor are upon the same plane and are of equal importance." Further, health reformers argued that the crowd-pleasing better baby contests stimulated local community interest in the health and well-being of children, resulting in "better children, better parents, and increased civic pride."[29]

On the other hand, the inherently competitive nature of these events also meant that baby contests were more likely to attract only those mothers whose children were already thriving. It is doubtful, for instance, that babies with congenital defects or chronic ailments would have been entered into competition at all, and it is uncertain how many entrants came from the most impoverished rural areas of the state where the population was much more likely to be malnourished or chronically ill. Thus, despite confident assertions by contest promoters that all rural mothers and children stood to benefit from the free health examinations and medical advice sessions these contests offered, giving out valuable health information within the context of an inherently competitive event seems a bit like preaching to the choir.

Contemporary appeals to community spirit aside, there remains the issue of the disturbing eugenic connotations underlying events that promoted the propagation of "better" babies. Conceptually rooted in the rural livestock show, contest promoters frequently made overt references to "raising good human stock" in publicizing the competitions. Indeed, in their attempt to draw in rural participants, event organizers seemed to take every opportunity to establish clear parallels between better baby contests and the livestock competitions that had already proven to be popular draws at agricultural fairs. The *Illinois Health News*, for example, made the link between livestock and human breeding quite explicit in its 1922 declaration that "No county fair is complete without provision to find the best human specimen (six months to five years of age) in the community, as well as the best hog, horse, sheep, etc." Further, the manner in which contestants were divided and classified raises a number of interesting questions about the ways in which health reformers and parents alike regarded physical and social differences among children.[30]

In addition to being grouped by age and sex, Illinois State Fair contestants were categorized by whether they lived in the country or the city; they also competed in special divisions designated for twins, triplets, and families of six or more children. A separate category for "colored" children appears intermittently in the Illinois State Fair records, although it is unclear whether the inconsistency reflects a decision to racially integrate the event at times or the fact that there simply were no nonwhite entrants in a particular year. Despite health officials' efforts to distinguish the events as "scientific" rather than mere beauty contests, examiners inevitably made subjective judgments about babies' facial or bodily features and apparent mental disposition or personality on the basis of their aesthetic and cultural preferences rather than on purely medical grounds. Racist attitudes on the part of contest organizers were commonly reflected in the stereotyped descriptions they entered on their scorecards. Historian Marilyn Irvin Holt has reported that judges in Riley County, Kansas, concluded that African American children suffered from defective diets despite the fact that over half their scores were at or above the average. Indeed, an extreme illustration of the racism underlying the early twentieth century's "better baby" movement may be found in the case of Elizabeth Tyler, a volunteer hygiene worker and baby contest organizer in Atlanta, Georgia, who in the 1920s became the first major female leader of the Ku Klux Klan.[31]

But, if the eugenic connotations of better baby contests are obvious, the precise nature of "eugenics" in the period under study here is itself a matter of considerable complexity. As historian Martin Pernick has argued, the scope of this rather amorphous discipline encompassed acquired as well as inherited diseases; state legislatures, for example, might include syphilis and tuberculosis among the disorders whose carriers could not marry under "eugenic" laws. Further, both scientific and popular understandings of the term "heredity" were quite broad in this era, and "passing on traits" to one's offspring had both environmental and biological meanings. Their efforts to judge country children separately from city children suggests that baby contest organizers tried to take into account the relatively poorer state of health that had been discovered among many rural children in Illinois. Publicity materials for better baby contests suggest that rather than endorsing the principle of selective human breeding, contest supporters instead attempted to dramatize the point that lifesaving hygiene and health care measures were under a mother's control; in essence, better health could be *learned*. In 1921, for example, public health officials proposed the addition of a ten-dollar prize for the "most perfect baby from each county" at the state fair; their objective in introducing this variation was that mothers would "take back to their communities the information obtained in regard to [the contests'] health educational benefits."[32]

Finally, although the event's popularity touched urban and rural settings alike in Illinois, health reformers deliberately attempted to draw upon the long-standing traditions of the agricultural fair in the belief that modern ideas about children's health care would be rendered more accessible, and perhaps more acceptable, to an audience of country dwellers. A range of competitive events already had been instituted at agricultural fairs in order to highlight rural women's talents in sewing, quilting, canning, baking, and handicrafts. Baby contest organizers in Illinois, eager to spread the message of modernization through better health among that state's rural fair-going population, promoted these events as a way to display, reward, and encourage the reproductive labors of women just as these fairs had by tradition celebrated the productive field accomplishments of farm men. "The Better Babies Contest is a comparatively new thing," declared the Illinois Farmers' Institute, "but it has come to stay just as the competition at fairs for cattle and grain and fruits have become a regular feature."[33]

Rather than "reducing" children's health care to the level of animal husbandry, the health reformers who promoted baby contests in this era intended to relay the message that the well-being of children was as vital to the interests of the rural community as was its economic interest in raising successful crops and healthy livestock; children's lives were valuable and worthy of the utmost public attention. An illustration that appeared on the cover of the March 1917 edition of *Illinois Health News* clearly reveals contest organizers' intentions in this regard (figure 4.2). In the cartoon, a whimsically rotund and happy baby holding a prize cup sits proudly among a cat, rabbit, dog, and chicken, each of which displays a first place ribbon. "A New Dignity for the Baby," the cartoon announced. "At last the Young Human Receives Consideration."

Popular campaigns to improve children's health in Illinois had gained considerable momentum by the time the First World War erupted in Europe. While Americans debated the pros and cons of preparedness for entering into the conflict, many reformers feared that the imperatives of fighting a war overseas would overshadow social welfare needs at home, including the provision of health education and services to women and children. Dr. Grace L. Meigs of the Children's Bureau had undertaken a study of the responses of child welfare reformers to the exigencies of wartime in several

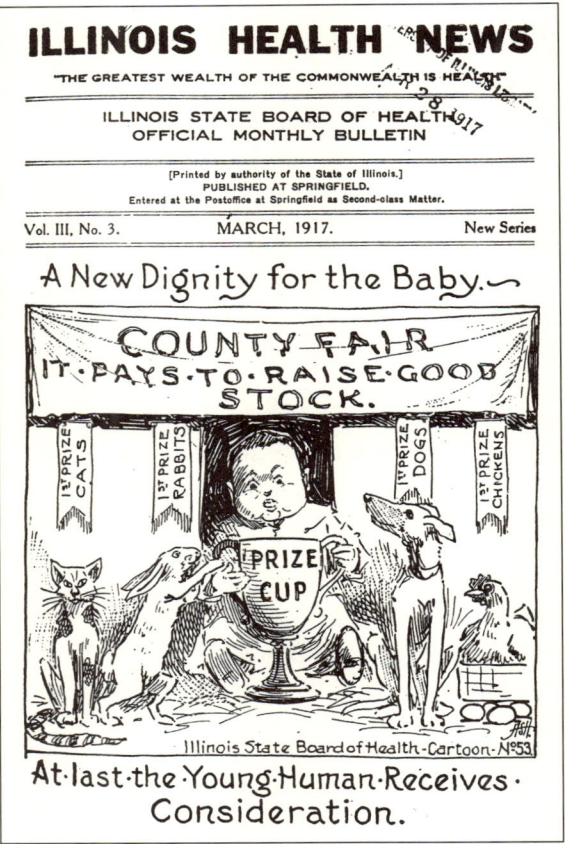

Figure 4.2. Cover illustration, *Illinois Health News* 3
(March 1917).

European nations. "If the experience of foreign countries is to teach us anything," she reported to her colleagues in the United States, "it should teach
us . . . that early in the war is the time to preserve the integrity of our work
for infant and maternal welfare, before that work is disorganized by the loss
of physicians and nurses. As the war goes on, doubtless many especial problems will arise."[34]

Heeding Meigs's warning, many health reformers in Illinois feared that
vital resources might be diverted to the war effort abroad; doctors and nurses
would be called to the front and therefore would be unavailable for public
health work at home. Chicago physician and child health advocate Caroline

Hedger, for example, had traveled to Belgium in 1915 under the auspices of the Chicago Woman's Club to work with typhoid victims among the civilian population there. *The American Journal of Public Health* pointed out that public health practitioners tended to be of draft age and encouraged communities to prepare for the possibility of losing their services. Further, husbands and fathers would be called for military service, and some reformers warned of the potentially negative health consequences for the women who would replace them working in dangerous war industries. "Mothers of young children under school age," cautioned Mary McDowell in the *Survey*, "working all night and having sleepless days — this is a challenge which cannot be ignored." Necessary sacrifices made in the cause of winning the war threatened to exact a high cost for the physical well-being of mothers and children.[35]

Other war-related concerns troubled health reformers as well. News from the front, some feared, would crowd out local publicity for various activities on behalf of public health. Chicago health reform advocates, in fact, had experienced just such frustration in April 1914, when the first baby week organized for the purpose of raising subscriptions to the Infant Welfare Society had taken place under a pall cast by the ominous political tensions that had erupted between the United States and Mexico. Despite widespread civic support (a sculpture of mother and child had been especially created for the event by the artist Lorado Taft), organizers were disappointed that the public's attention apparently had been diverted by the events in Mexico. "Instead of an elaborate campaign, daily luncheons, window displays and parades," the Infant Welfare Society reported with disappointment, "only one mass meeting took place in the Loop, on April 19th . . . The pages of the newspapers were filled with War instead of Charity, and where there had been dreams of hundreds of thousands of dollars, only $53,000 was secured." Because the Mexican situation had so thoroughly monopolized the public's attention, lamented the *Survey*, "so to all the other ravages for which war and the war spirit are responsible must now be added the needless deaths of Chicago babies."[36] The "war spirit" now being set loose throughout the country, it appeared, threatened to turn the American public's interest away from health and social welfare issues entirely. When in April 1917 American involvement in the war became a reality, reformers promoting health awareness and education among the general population were forced to both rethink and revise their strategies.

The National Council of Defense spearheaded a drive to form state-level councils for coordinating various home-front activities in support of the war effort. While the male-dominated councils took charge of finance, labor, and business issues, separate women's committees within each organization had "more to do with women and children and with the practical details of the home." A special Committee on Sanitation, Medicine, and Public Health was formed within the state's Council of Defense to help ensure that health standards on the Illinois home front would not deteriorate during the war. In May 1917 the heads of a number of women's organizations throughout Illinois met in Chicago's Orchestra Hall to form a Woman's Committee within the Illinois Council of Defense. The meeting attracted the talents of a number of prominent women reformers in Chicago. Jane Addams, representing the National Federation of Settlements, agreed to serve on the new committee's Advisory Council. Other council members included Chicago health and welfare activists Sophinisba Breckinridge and Alice Hamilton; Mary McDowell of the University of Chicago Settlement served on a special subcommittee on foreign-born women. The new committee saw its mandate as the coordination of all Illinois women's activities aimed at winning the war; the new Woman's Committee would serve as the nation's "second line of defense." Unity of purpose was to be the key to the committee's success; the war emergency required that all ideological differences, including those which had come to divide reformers themselves, be overcome. "I beg you to put aside all trivialities, all the unimportant things in life," the committee's chairwoman, wealthy Chicago reform activist and major Hull House benefactor Louise de Koven Bowen, urged, "and to dedicate yourselves solemnly to the task of winning the war."[37]

The new Woman's Committee that emerged within the Illinois Council of Defense represented an unprecedented concentration of the time and talents of hundreds of female volunteers who had already been active in a variety of causes throughout the state; the emergency of the Great War ignited a zeal for service among additional thousands of Illinois women who had not previously operated in the public sphere. Rather than allowing the war emergency to overtake the momentum in health and social welfare concerns, reformers instead established ideological links between their own causes at home and the war effort being waged abroad. In doing so, they gained in the Woman's Committee of the Illinois Council of Defense an efficacious and powerful new ally in carrying out their campaigns.

The first task was to register all available Illinois women for war work, and toward that end the Woman's Committee conducted a statewide census of all adult females available for civilian service, their special skills and pertinent experience, and the types of war service they were willing to perform.

Governor Frank O. Lowden urged that it was now time for Illinois women to put the talents they had perfected within their own homes and communities to work on behalf of the national interest. "There are a thousand activities for which women are particularly fitted," he announced, "and which will help greatly to maintain our morale in the field, and what is equally important, to maintain our morale at home." Leaving "nothing left undone, no stone unturned," the Woman's Committee's 2,136 local units enlisted a total of 692,229 women for war-related service, a figure representing nearly one-fourth of the state's entire adult female population. A number of counties reported that fully 100 percent of their women residents had been registered. This enthusiastic response on the part of civilian Illinois women became a source of extreme pride to the Woman's Committee. Publicity chairwoman Estelle Frances Ward declared in an essay published in the *Survey* that each Illinois woman's registration card served as a mirror "wherein she had a vision of her capabilities and shortcomings, and of her commercial and social value to the state." The large-scale mobilization of women into the war effort served to increase confidence in the worthiness of their own public activities as well as enhance their self-image as valued members of American society.[38]

Already well experienced in health and social welfare activism in Illinois, leaders of the new Woman's Committee determined that one of the most pressing home-front duties facing their newly mustered army was to conserve the health of children as a vital strategic measure for winning the war. Further, women's volunteer service in public health was all the more essential at this time, they argued, because so many trained medical professionals had been called to the colors, leaving "great gaps" in the "ranks of defenders of the health of the civilian population." In 1917, for example, forty-two staff members from the Visiting Nurse Association as well as the superintendent of the Infant Welfare Society left the Chicago area to serve overseas with the Red Cross. (Chicago residents would feel the absence of public health nurses acutely during the following year's influenza pandemic.)

But the important work of preventive health care and domestic hygiene instruction must not be forgotten in the wartime emergency, and the Woman's Committee endeavored to promote a "high standard of health, not as a humanitarian measure, but as a war measure"; members pledged to work toward the "elimination of waste in every phase of life." The needless deaths of children represented the most shocking waste of all, and certainly one that a nation at war could ill afford. Seizing the initiative, the Children's Bureau urged the formation of special child welfare departments within the defense councils that had been organized in each state. With the endorsement of President Woodrow Wilson — and an allocation of $150,000 from the federal wartime emergency fund — the bureau dispatched an urgent request for the cooperation of all councils in carrying out children's health campaigns as "a distinct war measure." Chicago-trained Julia Lathrop, the bureau's chief, made it clear that such efforts were not mere sentimental gestures on behalf of children, but rather represented key steps in an overall plan for conserving vital national resources while the nation was at war. The bureau called upon American women to save at least 100,000 of the 300,000 children who died annually in the nation. The quota for Illinois was set at 5,625 lives to be saved, and both Governor and Mrs. Lowden issued appeals to the people of Illinois to do their utmost to conserve the health of the state's youngest citizens.[39]

In January 1918 the Illinois Woman's Committee established a special Child Welfare Department charged with the task of "stirring up the State" to the necessity of conserving its children. "Women! Girls! What Are You Doing to Help Win the War?" exhorted a volunteer recruitment poster. Female citizens desiring to find their place in war work needed to look no further, for this poster also listed fifteen different ways in which Illinois women could serve their country on the home front. Topping the list was a patriotic appeal to join the crusade against infant mortality: "You can help save the babies for Uncle Sam." As de Koven Bowen observed, even school children had now become caught up in the excitement: "One boy wrote a composition in which he said, 'Now that we are at war, it is everybody's business to have a baby and to save it.'" The new Child Welfare Department received important financial backing from the Elizabeth McCormick Memorial Fund, a major supporter of innovative children's health activities in Chicago. Alice Wood, director of the fund, also served as chairwoman of the new Child Welfare Department. Wood was a seasoned veteran of health and social welfare efforts in Chicago and had served for seven years as president of the Illinois Training School for Nurses. Caroline Hedger, fresh from her work among typhoid fever victims in war-torn Belgium, was placed in charge of all children's health activities taking place in Chicago.[40]

The Child Welfare Department enjoyed the backing of numerous organizations in that city and throughout the remainder of the state. Its affiliates included a diverse amalgam of state and county agencies, private foundations, professional medical societies, labor organizations, and ethnic associations, all of which came together when the cause of preserving the lives of American children became refashioned into a war measure. Even the rather staid Infant Welfare Society of Chicago became caught up in the patriotic mood, revising the text of its normally sedate and tasteful publicity pamphlet and adding a jaunty new title, "Hold the Home Lines."[41] Within months the ambitious ideological mission of recasting the issue of health improvement for children in Illinois as a vital strategic measure for winning the war abroad appeared to have been largely accomplished.

But critical work remained to be done. In order to ascertain the status of child welfare activities already taking place in Illinois, the Child Welfare Department distributed questionnaires to health and social welfare organizations throughout the state. The department gathered information about the existence and number of baby clinics, day nurseries, public health nurses, and maternity hospitals; supervision of the local milk supply; medical inspections of schools; and plans for local baby week activities. Some of the data collected by the Child Welfare Department did in fact confirm health reformers' prewar fears. Many districts had indeed lost doctors and nurses to the front; some towns now had no physicians at all. One local chairman's answer to whether her district received the services of a school nurse was, "Yes, she visits once a year." Most rural counties in the downstate region remained without public health services of any kind. Members of the Child Welfare Department were surprised to discover that even the city of Chicago lacked sufficient facilities and equipment for carrying out public health activities at this time. When Caroline Hedger embarked on a program of weighing and measuring babies, for example, she found only seventeen infant scales in the entire city available for the task.

Clearly, then, existing resources would have to be shared among various health and social welfare organizations if the mandate to conserve children's health was to be carried out successfully. By working in cooperation with the Infant Welfare Society, the Visiting Nurse Association, the Department of Health, the Jewish Aid Society, and other service groups in the city, the Child Welfare Department was able to organize a number of infant health stations in schools, settlements, churches, and private club facilities in Chicago. As in the preventive health and hygiene campaigns of the prewar years, the education of mothers served as a key component of the wartime crusade. Convinced that "health instruction should be brought to the people where they naturally congregate," members of the Child Welfare Department conceived the inspired idea of establishing infant health stations at major Chicago department stores such as Marshall Field and Company and at such popular public attractions as the lion house in Lincoln Park Zoo.[42]

The issue of conserving children's health even entered into the martial atmosphere at the Chicago War Exposition. Public health and welfare exhibits had been held in that city for a number of years and such activities had regularly enjoyed widespread popularity among the general public. New to this 1918 exhibition, however, was the presentation of health reform as a distinct war measure. Public health nurses answered audience members' questions on preventive health and hygiene and gave baby care instructions to eager parents amidst the clamor of mock battles taking place outside the hall. Crowds of onlookers lined up to view a giant picture of General Pershing as a child, with the caption: "This is General Pershing at six years of age. Was it worth while to save this boy? He is helping to save the world." Although the Child Welfare Department originally had planned to bring in local children to serve as models in their health demonstrations, this measure proved to be unnecessary as crowds of mothers and fathers spontaneously handed their young ones onto the stage to be weighed and measured. The theme of working for health reform as a form of national war service was carried outside the exposition hall as well. Women volunteers staffing infant welfare stations, for example, were entitled to wear distinctive arm bands as "a special badge of honor, as long as service continued." Mothers bringing their babies for examinations at neighborhood health clinics received official window cards that featured Uncle Sam carrying a healthy baby on each shoulder; mothers were encouraged to display these emblems in their windows alongside Liberty Bond stickers to demonstrate their patriotism. But perhaps the most stirring demonstration of all came in the form of a Liberty Day parade held in Chicago that included among its numerous entries a float constructed by the Child Welfare Department. "Motherhood sat enthroned," one contemporary observer recounted, "surrounded by children of various ages, and holding the infant in her arms, while Uncle Sam stood at the rear, proud of his children and protecting the motherhood and childhood of the Nation. A boy scout at either side gave promise of future strength."[43]

In the patriotic zeal of wartime, interest in the preservation of health appeared to be at an all-time high. By directly linking the cause of health conservation with appeals to patriotism and national pride, Illinois health reformers had indeed succeeded in keeping their agenda alive on the home front. Infant welfare activities received unprecedented publicity as patriotic Illinoisans were exhorted to help Save the Babies for Uncle Sam in newspapers, posters, and pamphlets. "Communities which were unaware that they had a Child Welfare problem," the Woman's Committee reported with satisfaction, "have come to a realization that there is something to do for their

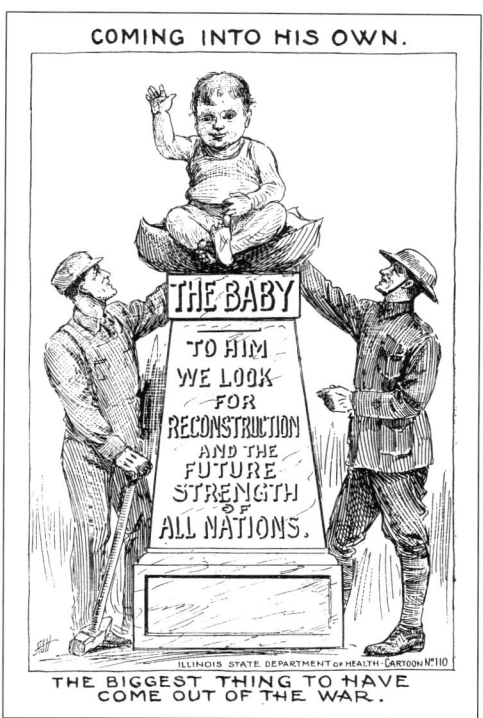

COMING INTO HIS OWN.

THE BABY

TO HIM
WE LOOK
FOR
RECONSTRUCTION
AND THE
FUTURE
STRENGTH
OF
ALL NATIONS.

ILLINOIS STATE DEPARTMENT OF HEALTH-CARTOON N° 110

THE BIGGEST THING TO HAVE
COME OUT OF THE WAR.

Figure 4.3. Cover illustration, *Illinois Health
News* 5 (July 1919).

children." By the war's end, volunteers in the Child Welfare Department
had weighed and measured babies in 1,261 localities throughout the state,
furnishing 338,719 special cards on which mothers could keep careful track
of their children's physical progress. Under the department's auspices, thirty-
seven new child health centers had been established, most of them located
in the Chicago area. Representatives from the Child Welfare Department
addressed over 500 public meetings on topics pertaining to infant and child
welfare in wartime. Illinois public health officials even went so far as to de-
clare the American baby "the biggest thing to have come out of the war."
Indeed, a 1919 cartoon in the *Illinois Health News* depicted an oversized
baby seated regally atop a pillar and flanked by masculine representatives of
labor and the military, both of whom looked up to the child as "the future
strength of all nations" (figure 4.3). In its final report the Woman's Committee declared that it had "helped to bring to the rural sections of Illinois the

truth of the statement that the children of the country are quite as much in need of care as those in the city, and in many cases, even more in need."[44]

In the wake of the unprecedented excitement generated by the wartime crusade, popular enthusiasm for "baby-saving" campaigns among both urban and rural residents of Illinois remained intense. The number of contestants entered in the better baby contest at the 1919 Illinois State Fair, for example, had more than doubled from the first such event held four years previously. Fully half of the exposition building at the fairgrounds was now taken up with examination rooms, a nursery, rest rooms, and a series of exhibits "showing a model nursery, sanitation methods, and other subjects of special interest to mothers." The "scientific" dimensions of the event itself had also been brought up-to-date, and the panel of judges now included two psychologists as well as medical doctors and a dentist. Even a statewide epidemic of polio in 1921 did not curtail popular enthusiasm for the better baby contest, and 831 babies found themselves being weighed, measured, and examined for defects at the state fair that year.[45]

As health reformers had hoped, small local fairs also proved to be an extremely popular venue for holding better baby contests, extending their modernization messages far into rural communities. In 1922, for example, a Kane County contest attracted over 400 participants, while another 300 babies came under the judges' scrutiny in the small central Illinois town of Paris. The *Prairie Farmer* even credited the addition of a contest featuring 375 infant competitors with the revival of local popular interest in the Champaign County Fair. In 1923, a total of seventy-nine such events were held in conjunction with local county and regional fairs in Illinois, with nearly 8,000 children entered into competition throughout the state.[46]

Unfortunately, maintaining an appropriate sense of decorum in the face of the baby contests' immense popularity with the general public presented its own set of challenges for event organizers. Illinois public health officials expressed alarm that many locally sponsored events had developed a tendency to "devolve into something of a show" in which the all-important health examinations were carried out in "such a superficial manner as to defeat the whole purpose of the conference." Every baby entered at a contest in the northern Illinois town of Aurora, for example, had been awarded a perfect score. Further, health officials sounded a warning that a "splendid opportunity for rendering a real service that will make for a sturdier citizenship and a general betterment of the public health" had largely deteriorated into a mere "display of children to the public and the exchange of expressions of parental pride." When the number of entrants neared one thousand at the 1922 Illinois State Fair, public health officials called for a special children's building to be installed at the fairgrounds. Convinced that the number of contestants had grown too large to serve the contest's educational mission — and worried that large crowds jamming the exhibition hall to view the proceedings posed a potential health hazard in and of themselves — public health officials attempted to limit the number of entries in the 1926 state fair. The scaled-down event disappointed fairgoers, however, and the following year the better baby contest was again "thrown open to as many as desired to come."[47] As an unparalleled public attention-getter and unmatched popularizer of children's health care, the better baby contest apparently was here to stay.

Also benefitting from all the wartime enthusiasm was the Illinois State Department of Public Health. Public health officials believed that the exigencies of the war emergency had served to justify the preventive health care and public education functions of this traditionally underfunded and politically unpopular agency. After the war, the department attempted to bolster its own weak apparatus by lobbying for legislation to provide a full-time health officer for every county in the state. Meanwhile, its popular education functions continued to expand. The department organized a series of "health pilgrimages," for example, in which its amassed resources were carried to rural communities, and three or four days of exhibits, lectures, and demonstrations on various public health topics were presented with the active participation of the local population. In addition to its now well-developed stock of pamphlets, display posters, and mechanical exhibits, the department was also making increasing use of the new medium of motion pictures to promote preventive health and hygiene education in a thoroughly modern way. By the 1920s the department's own rather extensive library of films contained titles produced by professional studios such as "The Man Who Learned" (Edison) and "The Long and Short Haul" (National). A film called "Tommy's Birth Certificate" promoted the proper registration of births while "The Priceless Gift of Health" contrasted the life stories of two boys, only one of whom had "grown up in hygienic conditions to healthy manhood." A film made by the Chicago production company Essanay entitled "Summer Babies" depicted the appropriate care of babies during the hot summer months "in a most entertaining manner." In 1921 a public health exhibit at the Illinois State Fair featured a specially constructed theater in which many of these films were screened for the fairgoing public.

The department made its film collection available to local community groups where their important messages reached audiences in small towns and rural communities. Red Cross nurses surveying health conditions in Macon County, in the central region of the state, described the vigorous response they received in one small town when they presented a film on the topic of children's health. Discovering that the community lacked a motion picture screen, the nurses, undaunted, showed the film by projecting it onto a sheet tied between two trees. "People came in their automobiles," one nurse reported, "and sat in them or on the ground and a great deal of interest and enthusiasm was shown." Following several major Hollywood scandals in the 1920s, commercial movie exhibitors in smaller communities increased their showings of health and hygiene films in an attempt to "relegitimate" filmgoing as a respectable leisure activity.[48]

Illinois health reformers faced the decade of the 1920s with considerable optimism. Popular health campaigns had been received by the public with enthusiasm among residents of cities, small towns, and rural areas alike, and a range of public and private organizations from the State Department of Public Health and the USDA's home extension services to local women's clubs had cooperated in health reform activities. Further, programs designed to bring modern and scientific preventive health and hygiene information directly to the people had received an unanticipated boost from the nation's entry into the Great War. The ideological reconstruction of health reform into a measure for winning the war had been, at least in the short term, a brilliantly successful strategy. Reformers had managed to keep the health needs of children squarely in the public eye at a time when attention and resources conceivably might have been diverted entirely to the imperative of waging war abroad. Instead, the grand vision of advancing social progress through improving the health of little citizens-in-the-making had been reimagined as a hard-headed and essential tactic for conserving a precious resource in a time of national crisis. After the war the Illinois State Department of Public Health, chronically underfunded and politically unpopular for decades, emerged a markedly stronger institution.

For their part, the grassroots women who supported public health efforts had fashioned an unprecedented public importance for their own volunteer activism as they stepped in to fill the health care gaps created when medical professionals left for war duties overseas. Caroline Hedger speculated about the more permanent possibilities of developing the grassroots network of female-led health care provision even further. "I would like to know," she ventured at a meeting of the American Association for Study and Prevention of Infant Mortality in 1918, "what the experts think about the possibility of training ordinary women, the kind of women that take home nursing courses under the Red Cross, the kind of women who by the war have been jolted out of their social activities, and what can be done in the training of those women to assist in the problem of breast feeding and the ordinary care of children in foreign neighborhoods?" Activists like Hedger experienced in wartime service what amounted to a revelation about the potential power held by grassroots women in the public life of Illinois.[49]

Historians interested in the American home front experience during the First World War have noted that the nationwide mobilization for the war effort provided a crucial testing ground for a number of progressive reform ideals, raising new and often puzzling questions about the appropriate relationship between public and private responsibility for matters of social welfare provision.[50] Likewise, the distinctive patriotic slant of the wartime health crusade in Illinois had cast a new light on the proper boundaries between the essentially private concerns of raising children and the very public business of ensuring a healthy and productive future citizenry as a matter of vital national interest. In his wartime representations, Uncle Sam had been depicted not only as exhibiting pride in his children, but as taking responsibility for their physical well-being as well. Thus an important, although largely unacknowledged, question underlay all the wartime exhibits, parades, and patriotic displays: If by bearing healthy children mothers provided the future strength and stability of the nation, then did the nation have reciprocal obligations for protecting the health and welfare of its mothers and children? Embedded within the wartime rendering of children's health conservation as a national goal was a subtler and more complex message that suggested a re-examining and perhaps even a redrawing of the perimeters delineating the private and public dimensions of health care provision in a modern society.

5

Contesting the Boundaries
of Health Care

P robably the largest delegation of women which ever appeared at the capital in support of legislation," the *Chicago Daily News* reported in
March 1923, "will be on hand . . . when the maternity and infancy bill is
discussed in joint public hearings this week or next." The occasion for this
gathering of female health reform activists in Springfield was a bill before
the state legislature authorizing the state to participate in the Sheppard-
Towner Act, one of the earliest federal social welfare measures enacted in
the United States. Approved by Congress two years earlier, the Sheppard-
Towner Act provided funds to individual states for the establishment of in-
structional programs in maternal and child health care. As the nation's leading child welfare organization, the female-led Children's Bureau had been
designated as the act's administering agency in Washington. To receive the
federal grants, the Children's Bureau required states to secure three things
from their own legislatures: official approval in the form of "enabling legislation," a designated agency to administer programs at the state level, and a
commitment of matching funds. Illinois health reform activists turned out
in full force in March 1923 as the General Assembly debated the pros and
cons of participating in the Sheppard-Towner program. Passage of maternity
and infancy legislation by Congress vindicated the long-held maternalist
position that safeguarding the physical well-being of mothers and children
must be made a top priority in the nation.[1]

Illinois health reformers were elated at the promise held out by the new
legislation. For years a broad coalition of public health practitioners, social
welfare advocates, and women's organizations had promoted preventive
health and hygiene education as both a private benefit and a public good.
Health reformers had long insisted that the eradication of preventable disease and untimely death in Illinois would serve as the very hallmark of a

120

modern midwestern state emerging from its benighted frontier past; declining rates of infant and childhood mortality had become important yardsticks by which to measure their state's social progress. Health reformers had exhorted thousands of mothers to exchange their unenlightened practices and superstitious beliefs for the modern, scientific principles of preventive health and hygiene.

Vibrant, diverse, and exceedingly popular with the public, health reform campaigns in both rural and urban areas of the state had gathered substantial momentum by the time the nation entered the First World War. The war itself threw the public dimensions of health care into sharp relief as a vigorous crusade led by the Woman's Committee of the Illinois Council of Defense urged the careful conservation of maternal and child health, not as a matter of philanthropy, but rather as a home-front strategy for winning the war. After the armistice, women's organizations, buoyed by the widespread popularity of wartime baby-saving activities, had continued their support of local preventive health activities. In February 1920, for example, the Woman's City Club of Chicago opened an infant welfare station at the corner of Osgood and Maude streets where an average of 150 children were weighed, measured, and examined each week. Later that year state public health officials credited the King's Daughters of Moline with reducing that city's infant mortality rates through their spirited preventive health and hygiene initiatives.[2] Illinois reformers viewed the Sheppard-Towner Act as an unprecedented opportunity to build upon the solid foundation laid down by years of state and local initiatives on behalf of maternal and child health.

The Illinois League of Women Voters (ILWV), headquartered in Chicago, emerged as the primary force behind this massive lobbying effort. Organized after the national women's suffrage victory in October 1920, the ILWV's stated purpose was to enable "women throughout the State to share actively in the formation of public opinion." Toward that end, the organization had been divided into several different committees, each designated to cover a specific topical area of legislation. The committees printed and distributed leaflets, conducted forums, issued press releases, and sent lobbyists to Springfield as well as Washington.[3] Significantly, many members of the ILWV enjoyed important connections to the Women's Joint Congressional Committee, the national organization that had used women's newly won voting power to successfully push for the passage of the Sheppard-Towner Act by Congress in 1921. A coalition of fourteen separate organizations including the Women's Christian Temperance Union, National Women's Trade Union League, Young Women's Christian Association, National Consumer's

League, the Medical Women's National Association, and the National League of Women Voters had waged what contemporary observers described as "the most intensive battle to influence the vote on a single bill that they had ever seen." In Illinois, Sheppard-Towner supporters' most influential link to this national maternalist coalition was the former chief of the Children's Bureau, Julia Lathrop, now serving as the ILWV's president. Although retired from her post in Washington, Lathrop maintained a regular correspondence with Grace Abbott, the Illinois health and social welfare activist who had succeeded Lathrop as the Children's Bureau chief.[4]

By the early 1920s, organized women's groups in Illinois had gained valuable experience in state-level political activism. Female suffragists had won women's right to vote in state-level elections in 1913; the "Illinois Law" amending the state's constitution went on to become a model for suffrage legislation in other states. Women's associations had secured the passage of a number of child welfare statutes in Illinois, including laws regulating child labor and the joint guardianship of children. In addition, they had acquired organizational and leadership experience during the First World War in the Woman's Committee of the Illinois Council of Defense. The campaign to secure enabling legislation for Sheppard-Towner represented one plank in a more ambitious political platform put forward by the ILWV in the postwar years that included support for an eight-hour work day for women, the exemption of mothers of young children from jury service, and the "representation of women by women on [political] party committees and in party conventions."[5] With the launching of its major campaign on behalf of Sheppard-Towner, the ILWV carried the progressive social reform goal of safeguarding maternal and child health squarely into the state's political arena.

Despite their initial high hopes, however, activists ultimately failed to translate widespread grassroots enthusiasm for preventive health campaigns into sufficient political clout for securing Sheppard-Towner programs in Illinois. A combination of competing political interests, the increasing commodification of preventive health care in the form of purchasable goods and services, and the waning power of maternalist ideologies in the 1920s came together to form a politically explosive mixture that crystalized in the contest over federally sponsored maternal and child health programs.[6] Ironically, Illinois maintained its position in the vanguard of health reform by becoming one of only three states (along with Massachusetts and Connecticut) that did *not* cooperate in the Sheppard-Towner program. Illinois's rejection of federally sponsored maternal and child health legislation signaled a sea change in the fortunes of progressive preventive health reformers nation-wide; the state went on to become a major player in securing the demise of the act at the national level as well. The Illinois debate over Sheppard-Towner reflects the changing context within which health reform campaigns operated in the 1920s as preventive health care moved more decidedly into the private realm of consumer goods and services. Diminishing in its func-tion as a social reform movement, the call to modernize mothers' role in preventive health care became more securely tied to the array of newly pur-chasable commodities that were becoming indispensable to the up-to-date household of the 1920s.

To Sheppard-Towner's supporters in Illinois, the new federal funds the act made available would serve as a major means for bolstering the state's notoriously sparse public health infrastructure, especially in rural areas. Even in medium-sized Illinois cities, expenditures for public health contin-ued to be meager. A 1919 survey by the Illinois Health Insurance Commis-sion, for example, revealed that the per capita dollar amount spent in Springfield stood at $0.13, less than one-fourth the amount spent annually in metropolitan Chicago.[7] A sweeping indictment of the inadequacy of public health services in that midwestern state capital had come in the form of a massive community survey undertaken by the Russell Sage Foundation in 1914. The survey's findings, published in 1920, gave eloquent testimony con-cerning the adverse health conditions endured by the poorest residents of the Illinois capital. Springfield's shockingly high infant mortality rates, for example, averaged approximately 127.4 deaths per 1,000 live births for the six years preceding the Russell Sage survey (1908–1913).[8]

The capital's 58,000 residents, the study revealed, were clearly segre-gated among the city's seven wards by income, race, and ethnicity. Although blacks and foreign-born whites constituted just over 19 percent of Spring-field's population, they formed 36 percent of the population in Ward 1 and 24 percent in Ward 6; each of these wards, located at the extreme eastern edge of the city, also contained larger proportions of infants and children. Strikingly, although these wards together accounted for 45.6 percent of all births in the city, they represented over 61 percent of all infant deaths. Even more disturbing was the fact that these deaths appeared to be from causes that public health reformers deemed to be largely preventable. Houses in Ward 1 were not connected to the city's water mains, for example, forcing some 11,500 residents to rely almost exclusively on wells and outdoor privies, a deplorable situation which, in the Sage Foundation's estimation, "put this section of the capital city of Illinois in a class with those small villages of the state which still depend upon the insanitary makeshifts of pioneer days." The close proximity of Ward 1 residents to each other rendered wells in this section of the city extremely hazardous, and the survey found that a "considerable number" of Ward 1 wells were indeed dangerously polluted. Interestingly, the survey also noted (but did not venture to explain) an unusually high incidence of premature births as well as stillbirths within these wards.[9]

Rates of illness from childhood diseases closely followed the striking pattern for infant deaths, with wards 1 and 6 containing the highest incidence of diphtheria, scarlet fever, whooping cough, and measles. Further, the survey discovered, eastside Springfield children were much more likely to die from these childhood diseases than were children in other sections of the city, a reflection of the distressing lack of medical care available to the city's poorest families. Noting the role of milk in spreading a number of contagious diseases, the surveyors deemed Springfield's milk supply to be especially objectionable, with little or no municipal regulation of rural suppliers and inadequate enforcement of the existing pasteurization codes.

Compounding the considerable health risks faced by Springfield's poorest residents was the lack of free or low-cost medical care available in the city. Except for a single dispensary operated by the Springfield Tuberculosis Association, there were no permanent free medical care establishments in the Illinois capital; free beds in the city hospital were available in the children's ward only. The city physician, an official appointed by the Sangamon County Board of Supervisors, remained obliged to treat all of the sick poor in the city in addition to providing medical supervision of the county and city jails. Remarkably, the city physician was also required to meet the cost of all prescriptions filled from his or her own modest stipend of one hundred dollars per month. "A more unsatisfactory system," declared the Russell Sage surveyors reproachfully, "could hardly be imagined."[10] Given these deplorable public health conditions, Sheppard-Towner supporters argued, preventive health and hygiene education for Springfield's poorest mothers and children constituted nothing short of an emergency measure.

The adverse publicity generated by the publication of the Russell Sage survey proved to be an important factor prompting the state's decision to reorganize its entire public health system in 1917. Just two years previously, a bill creating a special agency for children's health matters (modeled after the Children's Bureau in Washington) within the state public health department had been voted down by the Illinois General Assembly. In 1916, however, a major childhood polio epidemic visited the state and public criticism concerning the paucity of attention to children's health measures undoubtedly motivated many legislators to rethink their positions. The General Assembly approved the creation of a special child health division when it met again in 1917. The creation of this new bureau represented one relatively minor step in a year that saw a massive restructuring effort under Governor Frank Lowden in which virtually all of the state's various departments and agencies were to become more streamlined.

Importantly for supporters of preventive health work, the new public health department would no longer bear the obligation of licensing medical practitioners within the state, an extremely burdensome task which, according to one contemporary account, had been taking up fully 75 percent of the department's time and resources. As one of its last acts, the old State Board of Health had been instrumental in the passage of a new Medical Practice Act which substantially raised the professional education requirements for doctors, midwives, and other medical practitioners in Illinois. But, with the time-consuming responsibilities of regulating medical practice now going to a separate board, the reconstituted Illinois State Department of Public Health (ISDPH) became free to concentrate on designing and implementing policies and programs for advancing the public's health, for the first time becoming, in the words of director C. St. Clair Drake, a "Department of Health pure and simple."

A total of seven new specialized bureaus or divisions were created within the ISDPH, including one designated specifically to further popular health education through publications, exhibits, lecture services, and the increasingly used medium of motion pictures. Oversight of health initiatives designed especially for mothers and children would go to the new Division of Child Hygiene and Public Health Nursing. The new agency's mandate, Drake announced in an address given before the Illinois Public Health and Welfare Association in April 1917, was to "promote medical inspection of school children and . . . disseminate information and advice on the care of children."[11] With the organization of the new division, preventive health and hygiene education on the special behalf of Illinois children had become part and parcel of the state's public health structure.

In February 1921 Dr. Isaac D. Rawlings replaced C. St. Clair Drake as director of the ISDPH. A native of Illinois and graduate of Northwestern University's College of Medicine, Rawlings came to Springfield with more than twenty years' experience in public health work in Chicago, including playing a key role supervising the city's physicians during the devastating influenza pandemic of 1918.[12] Declaring that "the present system of local health administration is an insult to both the intelligence of the people and to any worth-while conception of public health service," Rawlings immediately launched an ambitious plan to bolster county-level public health work throughout the state. Under his new design, health commissioners in every Illinois county would oversee the conducting of sanitary surveys, develop and implement maternal and infant hygiene classes, and coordinate the various efforts of public and private health agencies within their own counties. Rawlings reportedly had found the inspiration for such a plan in the dynamic and popular local-level campaigns for both maternal and child health reform and tuberculosis prevention that had been waged throughout the state. His far-reaching proposal, however, went down to defeat in the Illinois General Assembly later that year. With deep regret the *Illinois Health News* informed its readers of "the failure of that progressive health measure . . . known as Senate Bill No. 294," a well-intentioned proposal that had "embraced the fundamentals for health promotion and disease prevention."[13] State resources for public health programs therefore remained scarce, and by 1922 the staff of the once-promising Division of Child Hygiene and Public Health Nursing consisted of only one superintendent, one assistant superintendent, a pediatrician, four nurses, and a stenographer. (Rawlings finally became exasperated when, in 1924, the division chief's post became vacant and only one applicant sought the job, a professionally humiliating situation that Rawlings himself blamed on the continued refusal of the state legislature to support the agency's work.)[14]

The Illinois General Assembly was not in session when federal Sheppard-Towner funding first became available in March 1922. Displaying dubious judgment, Governor Len Small gave his personal acceptance of the Sheppard-Towner program in the legislature's absence, apparently anticipating (incorrectly) that lawmakers would approve the required enabling legislation when they met the following year. The original bill had stipulated that states would receive a grant of $5,000 outright with an additional sum (the sum to be matched by the state) awarded according to the state's population as of the 1920 Federal Census. Under this plan Illinois, with a population of 6,485,280, stood to gain $14,631 for maternal and infant health programs. When added to the outright grant, the total Illinois appropriation for 1922 was $19,631. A check for this sum was duly delivered to the Illinois State Treasurer's office.[15] As the new director of the ISDPH, Dr. Rawlings had the duty of submitting the Illinois proposal for maternity and infancy programs to Grace Abbott, who had replaced Julia Lathrop as chief of the Children's Bureau. In a detailed letter to Abbott dated June 7, 1922, Rawlings outlined the scope of maternal and child health work to be performed in Illinois with Sheppard-Towner funds. Shoring up the state's weak public health apparatus, especially in areas outside of Chicago, represented the first priority listed under this proposal. The new Sheppard-Towner money, Rawlings explained, would be used to establish "infant, medical, and nursing activities in communities needing it, same to embrace all the surrounding rural districts."[16]

Under Rawlings's plan, public health nurses would take a leading role in carrying out the new maternal and child health programs he hoped to develop with Sheppard-Towner funds. At this time public health nurses in many rural areas provided nearly as broad a range of health services as did visiting nurses in American cities, including care of the sick, preventive health care instruction, prenatal and postnatal care and supervision, and school nursing.[17] A memorandum of agreement, drafted in 1920, had delineated the organization and supervision of all public health nurses in Illinois, including those employed by the newly formed Red Cross Town and Country Nursing Service, placing them under the ultimate supervision of the ISDPH. Despite the central role Rawlings planned for rural public health nurses in downstate maternal and child health work, however, they remained in exceedingly short supply; while an ISDPH directory recorded 396 public health nurses employed within the city of Chicago, only 102 were listed for the remainder of the state.[18]

Rawlings therefore proposed assigning public health nurses to entire counties, commissioning them "to locate and advise expectant mothers, and as early as possible refer the case to the family physician." Nurses would also oversee the distribution of educational literature on maternal and infant hygiene to all new and expectant mothers in their assigned counties. In addition, Rawlings planned to use Sheppard-Towner money to establish locally based infant welfare stations, modeled after the neighborhood well-baby clinics successfully operating in Chicago, in the downstate region. The staff at these stations would "diagnose ailments and refer [cases] to physicians, instruct [mothers] in feeding and handling of infants, disseminate knowledge in maternal and infant care to both physicians and the public, [and] prescribe infant feeding modifications whenever the patient is unable to secure the services of a private physician." Finally, the ISDPH's infant welfare staff also would follow up on all special needs cases brought to their attention.[19]

Although Rawlings's plan put forward definite ideas about how to utilize Sheppard-Towner funds in Illinois, he also expressed anxiety about securing the required state matching funds from the General Assembly. Rawlings compiled a list of the various monies that could be pooled from existing ISDPH resources in order to meet the state funding requirement at the outset. "There seems to be no other way to match the Sheppard-Towner funds," he explained to Abbott, "until such time as the Legislature can be given an opportunity to provide funds for the biennium beginning July 1923 if they wish to do so."[20] Rawlings had good reason to be wary. Several bills to raise taxes in order to finance the matching requirement had already reached the Illinois General Assembly, even before the passage of the Sheppard-Towner Act by Congress. Each bill, however, had died in committee. To make matters worse, the Illinois attorney general decided that the scandal-plagued Governor Small, in fact, had acted illegally in accepting the funds forwarded from the Children's Bureau; the federal money, he concluded, could not be accepted by the governor without the authorization of the state legislature. Thus, Illinois found itself unable to use the initial appropriation it received from the Children's Bureau in 1922. The following year, the first full year that the Sheppard-Towner Act came into effect, Congress designated a total of $950,000 for division among the participating states. Illinois's share stood at $48,739; this, then, became the target sum to be matched from the state budget.[21] The lobbying campaign to secure the prerequisite legislation from the General Assembly now began in earnest.

On June 21, 1922, the ILWV sponsored a general meeting of Chicago-area women activists to discuss a strategy for bringing Illinois into compliance with the Sheppard-Towner Act. A number of child health and welfare organizations throughout the city sent representatives to the meeting, including the American Red Cross, Infant Welfare Society, Chicago Lying-In Hospital, Chicago Industrial Nurses' Club, and the Illinois Federation of Women's Clubs. Dr. W. A. Evans, a hygienist who had acted as the main force behind Chicago's mandatory milk pasteurization ordinance in 1909 and now served on the state's Board of Public Health advisors, presented the Rawlings plan for using the anticipated Sheppard-Towner funds. The updated plan now included a campaign for improving birth registration throughout the state as well as reorganizing the department's child hygiene work in order to place more emphasis on preventive health functions, including prenatal and newborn services.[22] Evans expressed concern that securing both the required enabling legislation and the matching grant from the state legislature might prove politically difficult. He advised Sheppard-Towner supporters attending the meeting that special emphasis should be placed on garnering the support of businessmen and small farmers, groups that had allied on a number of previous occasions to oppose the expansion of state government in Illinois. Evans did not foresee the potential for opposition from physicians in the state, and in any case he discouraged attempts "to convert the doctors as they do not wield much influence." Sara Place of the Infant Welfare Society, however, disagreed, arguing that it was "not wise to neglect the family physician as most parents of children would be apt to accept his version of the soundness of the Act and if he were against it or indifferent to it, it would be difficult to persuade men to support it." Unfortunately for supporters of Sheppard-Towner in Illinois, Evans's own assessment of his colleagues' response to maternal and child health legislation proved to be politically naive.[23]

Sheppard-Towner proponents developed a two-pronged approach to secure support for their cause. First, they would demonstrate to the public a clear need for federal funding to fight the high rates of maternal and child mortality that still plagued some parts of the state. Averaging state public health data for 1920 and 1921, for example, proponents discovered that ten counties in Illinois still had infant mortality rates greater than 100 per 1,000 live births. (Infant mortality in Cook County, by comparison, had fallen to 88.1; the figure for Chicago stood at 89.3).[24] The First World War infant mortality crusade, moreover, had demonstrated the high public relations value of promoting maternal and child health reform as an *emergency* measure, one so severe that it appeared to require immediate federal assistance. "I believe Act #1 should be introduced first and pushed forward as fast as possible," Rawlings wrote to Edith Rockwood of the ILWV. He urged that the legislation include an emergency clause "so we get these funds now past due as soon as possible and get busy with Sheppard-Towner activities."[25] Second, proponents of enabling legislation established that the kinds of programs that Sheppard-Towner would fund — maternity and infancy education, locally based well-baby centers, nurse-advisors for new mothers — represented the best means for improving the health of mothers and children in Illinois.

Using data from the ISDPH, proponents found that six of the ten counties with the highest infant mortality rates in the state currently had no public health nurse, while none had an infant welfare center. Conversely, of the seventeen counties that did have infant welfare centers, fourteen had infant mortality rates below the state average.[26] Sheppard-Towner backers set out to convince the citizens of Illinois that there existed a clear causal link between the local availability of maternal and infant health programs and lower infant mortality rates in the state. Once such a connection was established in the public mind, they theorized, political support for the legislation

would naturally follow. In November 1922 proponents formed a special steer-
ing committee, the Joint Committee for the Maternity and Infancy Bill, for
the purpose of "organizing the expression of opinion." Alice Wood, representing the Elizabeth McCormick Memorial Fund, was appointed chair of
the new committee. Wood, the director of the wartime infant mortality campaign in Illinois, seemed an apt choice for the job. She urged the various
organizations working to promote Sheppard-Towner throughout the state to
pool their information and produce a single, comprehensive, and accessible
public relations document explaining the desirability of securing federally
sponsored maternal and child health programs in Illinois. The organizations
responded to Wood's call, and the resulting pamphlet entitled "A Much
Needed Service for Mothers and Babies" emphasized the urgency of establishing Sheppard-Towner programs in Illinois and described a range of activities that could be sponsored with federal funding.[27]

But, as Sheppard-Towner advocates were soon to learn, a political
change was in the wind. Although in previous years the goal of advancing
social progress through disseminating modern methods of preventive health
and hygiene had served as a unifying theme among a diverse range of groups,
by the early 1920s many in Illinois had become alarmed by the unprecedented role created for government by the Sheppard-Towner Act. As an organizational model, designers of the federal maternity and infancy program
had looked to the Smith-Lever Act that since 1914 had provided federal aid
for state-run programs in agricultural research and education. Advocates of
Sheppard-Towner in Illinois hoped to duplicate the success of the U.S. Department of Agriculture's farm and home extension services in the state; the
county-based, private/public cooperative system of Farm and Home Bureaus
had continued to flourish in Illinois after the war.

Under the terms of the Sheppard-Towner Act, each state was required
to submit to the Children's Bureau a set of detailed plans for funding, designing, and implementing maternal and child health programs. These individual state plans remained subject to the approval of a federal board which
consisted of the chief of the Children's Bureau, the Surgeon General of the
United States Public Health Service, and the United States Commissioner
of Education. The state, for its part, would be granted complete authority in
designating an administering agency, establishing the mechanics of implementation, and developing the actual programs to promote maternal and
child health education. The act's supporters frequently pointed to the successful precedent already set by joint federal and state funding for the establishment of land-grant colleges, the rehabilitation of war veterans, and the
expansion of the state highway system.

Others, however, viewed this trend with dismay. Coming before Congress to oppose the Sheppard-Towner Act in 1921, the Civic Federation of Chicago testified that the "tendency to extend Federal subsidies to local governments is unsound fiscal policy leading to extravagance in local government, demands for increasing Federal aid, and greater tax burdens."[28] In a 1923 editorial the *Chicago Daily News* warned of the growing dangers of government paternalism, asserting that "anything that weakens the self-reliance of the individual or the community is a direct invitation to dependence and the servile attitude that goes with it. . . . Acceptance of doles from federal authority is both humiliating and demoralizing. This state cannot stoop to mendicancy without suffering the inevitable consequences."[29] To its detractors in Illinois, the Sheppard-Towner Act represented the thin end of a wedge prying open a Pandora's box of future paternalistic ventures on the part of the federal government. Modernity must come to Illinois, they insisted, but not at the expense of individual initiative and states' rights.

Leadership of the anti-Sheppard-Towner forces in Illinois, however, came not from that state's business leaders but rather from physicians in private practice. Following the act's passage by Congress, the Illinois State Medical Society (ISMS), an organization of about 7,000 members, sounded a clarion call over what it perceived to be the encroaching power of government in the provision of health care. As public health activities had proliferated in Illinois, physicians in private practice had come to see their own interests as allied more closely with those of increasingly regulated industrialists than with maternalist social reformers. Along with their allies in business, doctors argued that both state and federal government largesse had grown out of control in the years since the First World War and must be kept in check. The business-medical alliance in Illinois fought against a range of social welfare measures in this period, including compulsory health insurance, the eight-hour workday for women, workmen's compensation, and the national child-labor law.[30]

The Sheppard-Towner Act placed too much responsibility in the hands of the state for matters pertaining to the health and welfare of American children, they argued, matters that by tradition had remained more appropriately circumscribed within the boundaries of the private family. "The Constitution gives Congress power to 'raise and support armies' and the duty of caring for the 'Nation's defender, his widow and orphans,' as Lincoln said," the ISMS's official organ, the *Illinois Medical Journal*, insisted in 1921. "But the Constitution does not give Congress power to raise and support children, nor the right to tell states and parents how they shall be reared." Conservative objection to the bill's original wording had led to the attachment of a proviso stipulating that "the plans of the States under this Act shall provide that no official, or agent, or representative in carrying out the provisions of this Act shall enter any home or take charge of any child over the objection of the parents, or either of them, or the person standing in loco parentis or having custody of such child."[31]

Organized physicians had begun honing their political skills during a fierce nationwide campaign against compulsory health insurance waged by the American Medical Association (AMA), headquartered in Chicago. In 1917 the Chicago Medical Society joined forces with the ISMS in an aggressive campaign to get a bill proposing state-sponsored health insurance for all persons earning less than $100 per month defeated in the Illinois General Assembly. The allied physicians' organizations then went on to take an active role in opposing compulsory health insurance on the national level as well. This crucial political victory subsequently emboldened the AMA to vigorously oppose any form of "state medicine," a term the organization applied to any program of health care provision or education that involved the participation of local, state, or federal government entities.[32]

The maternal and child health education programs proposed under the Sheppard-Towner Act were to be supervised ultimately by the Children's Bureau, a nonmedical agency within the U.S. Department of Labor, and thus its opponents contended that Sheppard-Towner represented an unwarranted and perhaps even unconstitutional intrusion by the federal government into private medical practice in their state. (Like-minded activists in Massachusetts mounted an unsuccessful challenge to the constitutionality of the Sheppard-Towner Act in the United States Supreme Court.)[33] In 1921 the president of the ISMS, Dr. Charles E. Humiston, appeared before a congressional committee to outline Illinois physicians' objections to the pending maternal and infant health bill. When Congress nevertheless passed the measure, Humiston responded by writing an official resolution against Sheppard-Towner adopted by the AMA at its annual meeting in May 1922.[34]

By the time the Sheppard-Towner bill came before the Illinois General Assembly in 1923, doctors in private practice had already entered into a fierce battle for professional control over the relatively new field of preventive health care. On the one hand, many general practitioners in both urban and rural areas of the state perceived themselves to be losing ground to younger physicians trained in relatively new medical specialties such as obstetrics and pediatrics. On the other hand, the provision of preventive health care represented a new practice field in the 1920s, one that had been pioneered primarily not by medical doctors but by progressive social workers, educators, public health nurses, nutritionists, and child welfare advocates. After the

First World War, Illinois doctors — somewhat belatedly — sought to gain control over this growing segment of the health care field.[35]

Although physicians in private practice had commonly teamed up with public health practitioners in Progressive Era health reform campaigns, the emergence of a larger, stronger state department of public health in 1917 disturbed many medical doctors in Illinois. In 1920 the ISMS passed an official resolution condemning the principle of state aid in health work as "pernicious and dangerous . . . an encroachment on the functions of the State and an invasion of State authority tending to the demoralization of State Public Health work, rather than its development." Alarmed that the medical profession seemed to be coming under siege in their state, Illinois delegates to the AMA's annual meeting in 1920 were instructed to "oppose state medicine, compulsory health insurance, county and state health agencies, and allied dangerous Bolsheviki schemes."[36] Increasing numbers of Chicago physicians in private practice voiced their resentment over the proliferation of free clinics and neighborhood dispensaries in their city. In the wake of health reformers' well-intentioned but rather misguided efforts to provide health care to the deserving poor, they charged, patients who were perfectly capable of paying for a visit to a doctor's office were now instead "abusing" the services offered at free and low-cost clinics. In March 1921 the ISMS announced that a new survey of Illinois physicians had clearly demonstrated that the public health centers being advocated by health reformers for the downstate region were not in fact needed. (The general public, as potential clients of such services, had not been queried on this question.)

In response, the Chicago Community Trust published a report the following year countering that patients were not in fact overusing dispensaries in that city, at least not for prenatal care. "Antenatal examination and care involve too much that is intimate and personal to make clinics sought unless needed," the report asserted. "Until long past the time that the present number of prenatal clinics in Chicago are used to their limit, there will be no real problem of their abuse by prospective mothers."[37] After years of working to convince immigrant women to abandon the services of unlicensed midwives, apothecaries, healers, and quack doctors and to utilize "modern, American" health care instead, reformers saw increased attendance at local facilities as a cause for celebration rather than lament. The argument over patients' use and abuse of free clinics continued unabated throughout the decade of the 1920s.

Some Chicago physicians in private practice resented the central role played by the Visiting Nurse Association (VNA) in providing preventive health care services in that city. As their popularity with their poor and working-class clientele spread and their caseloads significantly increased, VNA nurses began to walk a rather fine line between providing much-needed health care to underserved immigrant and African-American populations and stepping on the professional toes of Chicago's politically powerful doctors. The nurses' sensitivity to their own position is reflected in the VNA's training manual, which included lessons in professional etiquette. When visiting a home for the first time, the manual instructed, nurses must ascertain first that no physician was already attending the case and second that the family was truly unable to pay for a local doctor's services. If a nurse determined that a particular situation required the attention of a medical specialist, she was directed to approach local physicians about providing the services free of charge, but only after a careful consideration of the merits of the case. "Before asking too much time from a busy man," the manual advised, "talk over such cases with your Supervisor."[38]

Despite such careful attention to professional protocol, however, public health nurses found themselves increasingly under attack by the ISMS. Nurses providing health care services in that state's public schools, for example, were accused by the ISMS of illegally practicing medicine: "The nurse is extending an authority of her license," the *Illinois Medical Journal* argued in 1920, "if not actually violating the law regulating the practice of medicine." But the journal went even further, jealously charging that under the rubric of health reform "nurses have been lauded and cajoled to such an extent that they not only feel that they are an indispensable factor in public health service, but that they are really the whole thing and that the service would be much better off if the physicians would withdraw and leave the field to them."[39] The central role for public health nurses in the maternal and child health programs envisioned under Rawlings's plan greatly exacerbated these professional tensions.

Such unbridled hostilities expressed in the official organ of the state's most important medical society exemplified an aggressive backlash against the Progressive Era's assumptions about the meaning of health care. In the absence of therapeutic measures to cure most diseases once they had been contracted, progressive health reformers had argued that disseminating modern, scientific preventive health and hygiene information as widely as possible represented the best hope for improving the nation's standard of well-being. Raising the levels of education and training for all women, they had insisted, would bring modernity to Illinois by facilitating the acculturation of immigrant communities and uplifting agrarian life. Visiting nurses, public health officials, social workers, women's club members, and agricultural extension agents had united in their efforts to modernize the way Illinoisans ate, drank, bathed, slept, kept house, worked, and gave birth. Reformers intended the new programs under Sheppard-Towner to build upon this foundation, with the bulk of maternal and child health work to be carried out by public health nurses, social workers, and other practitioners of preventive health care.

Both the Children's Bureau and Sheppard-Towner backers in Illinois had repeatedly insisted that, because such activities disseminated valuable preventive health care information to mothers who otherwise lacked access to the services of private physicians, they were actually *complementary* to the practice of medicine, not in competition with it. Physicians claiming the new field of preventive health care for their own, however, contended that dispensing maternal and infant health care advice to women actually constituted practicing medicine, and thus should remain solely in the hands of medically trained and state-licensed physicians. The Illinois physicians who opposed Sheppard-Towner charged that maternal and child health programs were nothing short of irresponsible because they allowed the crucial role of patient educator to rest in the hands of "lay" people, i.e., nurses, teachers, social workers, and midwives. In his testimony before the House committee in 1921, Dr. Humiston put this argument squarely before Congress:

> The mother and the prospective mother, with her new babe need the best scientific instruction; not merely non-technical instruction. . . . where would you look for that except among those who have dedicated their lives to acquiring and giving that kind of instruction?. . . . This is a medical question, it is supervising the practice of medicine in the different states through a Children's Bureau in the Department of Labor that this bill provides. That is why we object to it. . . . We object to placing the practice of medicine or any part of it under the supervision of a lay board.[40]

While all sides in the debate over Sheppard-Towner in Illinois could agree that the modern precepts of preventive health and hygiene represented the best means for safeguarding maternal and child health in their state, the issue of who would *control* this vital information had become bitterly contested ground.

In the first weeks of 1923, the coalition supporting Sheppard-Towner intensified its efforts in anticipation of the reconvening of the Illinois General

Assembly later that spring. A Chicago-area law firm drafted the text of the bills to enact enabling legislation in the General Assembly, with identical language for both the House (H. B. 298) and Senate (S. B. 175) versions. The bills provided for the acceptance of the Sheppard-Towner Act by the State of Illinois, designated the ISDPH as the agency to carry out the act's provisions in the state, authorized the State Treasurer to act as custodian of all monies allotted to the state from the Children's Bureau, established a "Federal Aid Maternity and Infant Hygiene Fund," and authorized the Auditor of Public Accounts to draw warrants upon the fund. Reflecting proponents' strategy of promoting maternal and child health measures as a matter of extreme urgency, the final section of the bill proclaimed that "because of an emergency this Act shall take effect upon its passage."[41]

Once the bills were drafted, the ILWV then devoted considerable attention to choosing the bills' sponsors in the General Assembly. When approached on the topic of strategy by the ILWV, Illinois House Speaker Shanahan recommended that the "chief consideration in choosing a proponent for the bill was his or her interest, a person who would not put the bill in 'by request,' someone who would push it thru [sic] his or her own initiative." Further, in order to maximize the bill's chances for success in the legislature, its sponsors in both houses clearly must be from the Republican Party, as the Democrats had controlled the Illinois General Assembly for a total of only four years between 1880 and 1923.[42] One promising possibility was William G. Thon, a Cook County Republican who formerly had served as chair of the Committee on Charities and Corrections; Shanahan found him to be "a good man but very busy." Dr. Grace Meigs of the Children's Bureau telephoned the ILWV's headquarters in Chicago to recommend Thomas J. Hair of the Fifth Senatorial District: "He is a university graduate, is young, energetic, is just the kind of person we should like to have behind the bill." Further, Meigs promised to use "whatever influence she had" in securing his support. In February, however, the Joint Committee reported to the ILWV that Thon and Joliet Republican Richard J. Barr had agreed to sponsor the bills.[43]

With this critical support in Springfield assured, then, members of the Joint Committee lobbied hard over the next several months. They adopted the tactic of buttonholing individual state legislators whenever and wherever possible and recording the responses they received on index cards, which were then kept on file at ILWV headquarters. (This particular system apparently greatly irritated Sheppard-Towner opponents, who referred to the practice pejoratively as "card-indexing.") The responses that lobbyists recorded on their index cards ranged from the carefully formulated answer of Representative Hair ("I am in favor of all measures to properly promote the welfare and hygiene of maternity and infancy"), to the firm, unconditional resistance of Representative Frank A. McCarthy of Elgin ("Opposed"), to the noncommittal and politically ambiguous reply offered by Representative Thomas Johnson of Streator ("We always stand for better manhood and womanhood.")[44]

Through their energetic efforts proponents of Sheppard-Towner succeeded in garnering at least some support in quarters that at the outset had been less than assured. The bills to enact enabling legislation received the "hearty backing" of Illinois labor organizations, for example, a group that had remained conspicuously aloof from the earlier battle over compulsory health insurance. The act's supporters were elated at this nod of support from labor. In a report to Alice Wood of the Joint Committee, lobbyist Julia Scott Vrooman described with a note of triumph her experience in collaring Representative Martin Brennan of Bloomington at a train station: "I emphasized the fact that all our local labor organizations had gone on record as favoring the bill — which gave him decided pause, as he looks for support in that quarter." In addition to labor, several prominent religious organizations in the state also came on board in support of Illinois's participation in the new maternal and child health program. Although in Massachusetts Roman Catholic groups had opposed Sheppard-Towner as an unwarranted intrusion by government into the sanctity of the private family, the Chicago branch of the National Council of Catholic Women backed enabling legislation in Illinois and the *New World*, the official organ of the Chicago Archdiocese, published editorials in support of the act.[45]

Women in rural downstate Illinois represented a crucial source of support for the bill soon to come before the General Assembly, for farm women potentially had the most to gain from Sheppard-Towner legislation. As the federal-level administrators of the act, child health advocates within the Children's Bureau may have found an especially receptive audience among the white, native-born women who represented the overwhelming majority of the rural female population in Illinois. What is more, the editors of a number of progressive farm journals clearly perceived that their readers' interests would be served by the Sheppard-Towner Act. The influential farm women's magazine *The Farmer's Wife*, for example, had supported the bill when it came before Congress in 1921.[46]

By the 1920s, rural areas throughout the United States were receiving much less assistance from public and private child health and welfare agencies than were the major cities. Many reformers not only saw a greater need for federally sponsored health programs in the countryside, they also believed that public health clinics operating in more remote areas where doctors were relatively scarce would pose less of a threat to physicians in private practice. Deficient of public health services, the rural downstate region of Illinois also lacked the benefit of child health and welfare programs sponsored by private charitable and philanthropic organizations, which had formed an important part of health reform efforts in Chicago. Indeed, a 1922 Children's Bureau directory of child health agencies in Illinois lists only nineteen such agencies (both public and private) for communities outside of Chicago, and only *one* rural child health agency operating in the state, the Vermilion County Tuberculosis Association.[47]

Sheppard-Towner funds, therefore, would prove most useful of all in supporting the initiation and development of maternal and child health work in rural Illinois. Further, Illinois farm women were likely to regard the type of private/public cooperative venture that Sheppard-Towner represented to be the most appropriate means for carrying out rural health reform efforts. For a number of years, farm women had been actively participating in the USDA's home extension services established by the Smith-Lever Act, the model for Sheppard-Towner. The Home Bureaus, in fact, became among the most important organizations carrying out public health work in the downstate region. It is not surprising, then, that in 1923 women in the Illinois Farmers' Institute gave enabling legislation for Sheppard-Towner their warmhearted approval at the annual meeting of the Institute's Household Science Department in Belleville (near St. Louis). The members recognized that "the mortality of mothers and children is still high, and higher in our rural communities than among [the] urban population." They went on to acknowledge that this situation was due at least in part to rural mothers' lack of knowledge concerning "the rules of hygiene governing the prenatal period and care of the young child." The women, therefore, urged the state legislature to meet the federal requirements for participation in the Sheppard-Towner Act.[48]

Last, but by no means least important to Sheppard-Towner supporters in Illinois, was the delicate task of garnering support for their cause among the various medical organizations in the state. The Chicago Pediatric Society, for example, came out in favor of enabling legislation. Dr. Joseph DeLee, founding director of the Chicago Lying-In Hospital and an influential figure in Chicago medical circles, also strongly endorsed Sheppard-Towner in a letter to Alice Wood: "I am heartily in favor of any movement whose object is to better the condition of the child-bearing women of the United States."[49] A group of twelve Chicago-area doctors produced a pamphlet putting forth their own support on behalf of Sheppard-Towner. The group, which included health reform activists Caroline Hedger and W. A. Evans, asserted that the kind of educational programs to be funded represented an effective means of combatting high rates of maternal and infant mortality because "ignorance of the mother in child care raises death rates as well as does lack of care or improper care at maternity and poor, or no, nursing."[50] Copies of the pamphlet were distributed by the ILWV. In addition, Alice Wood of the Joint Committee sent a letter to the presidents of a number of medical organizations throughout the state urging them to "talk to [their] own physicians. Try to win their favor for the bill. Some doctors are against it because they have been misinformed of the purposes of the act, and we find very few of them have read the original bill."[51] Wood's comments proved insightful, for while a number of individual physicians did in fact back Sheppard-Towner legislation in Illinois, the medical profession as a whole was anything but unanimous in its support.

Meanwhile, the coalition opposing Sheppard-Towner had also worked hard to make its objections heard. Business and civic leaders raised the issue of fiscal responsibility in an age of burgeoning government largesse. Those who worried about the undesirable fiscal and social ramifications of Sheppard-Towner also made the more utilitarian argument that the monetary award the state would receive under the terms of the act fell far short of the amount actually rendered to the federal government by Illinois taxpayers. Poorer states, they insisted, stood to gain at the expense of Illinois. Douglas Sutherland, secretary of the Civic Federation of Chicago, asserted that the appeal of federal aid "is strongest to the less populous states, because they will get more out of the 'pot' than they put into it." A *Chicago Tribune* editorial cautioned that Illinois would receive $58,739 under the act while its citizens would actually pay out $125,363 in federal taxes. Even more state taxes would be levied in the future, they argued, to meet the matching-funds requirement. "The tendency to delude ourselves into the belief that we are getting something for nothing," the editorial continued, "and the tendency to crowd more and more improper functions upon the federal government are serious evils. They must be fought." (Such arguments by Sheppard-Towner opponents prompted Julia Lathrop to suggest that the ILWV organize for its own members "an elementary course in Illinois taxation and expenditure.")[52]

No source proved to be more vociferous in its opposition to Sheppard-Towner, however, than the *Illinois Medical Journal*, the official organ of the ISMS. The journal denounced the Sheppard-Towner Act relentlessly, from the time of its inception until that legislation's eventual demise in 1929. Because it believed that the act posed a menace to the integrity of the entire medical profession, the *Journal*, under the editorship of Dr. Charles J. Whalen, did not confine its attentions solely to developments in the state of Illinois, but rather fought on for the repeal of Sheppard-Towner at the national level as well. "It is a wholly Prussian idea that the state has more knowledge than all its citizens, and can only lead to disaster," one typical Whalen editorial forewarned. (Opponents of state-sponsored medical programs in this era commonly labeled them "Prussian" because Germany had passed the first compulsory health insurance law in 1883. During the anti-German hysteria of the First World War rumors had arisen that health insurance was a kaiser-inspired plot to spread German *Kultur* to the United States.) Alternately, the *Illinois Medical Journal* also declared that "when the 150,000 physicians, 220,000 nurses and 2.400,000 annual mothers [sic] depend for instruction and advice on a single political bureau at Washington, America will be another failure like Rome and Russia." Whalen, a graduate of Rush Medical College in Chicago who later became a faculty member there, had also obtained a Bachelor of Law degree from Northwestern University.[53]

In his consuming zeal to see Sheppard-Towner defeated, Whalen was not above reprinting articles from ultraconservative organizations that bordered on hysteria. One piece, reprinted from the Massachusetts Civic Alliance, put the case against Sheppard-Towner in no uncertain terms: "Maternity legislation is paternalism, communism, sovietism, and all the isms of the kind condensed into one." The author went on to warn ominously that government sponsored maternity programs would result in the "placing of American mothers and their children under departments of governments, where cattle are placed, and, in some respect, for the same purposes." Another article, reprinted from the *Woman Patriot*, inexplicably accused William Randolph Hearst of lurking behind the Sheppard-Towner Act and asked its readers, "Will the Hands of Hearst rock the cradle and the ship of state?"[54] Whalen's diatribes on the editorial pages of the *Illinois Medical Journal*, of course, cannot be considered representative of the views of all physicians in Illinois, or even all members of the ISMS. At the same time, however, Whalen's colleagues tacitly gave approval to such invectives by not openly challenging his editorship of the journal during his long tenure there. The rather enigmatic political views Whalen expressed in his frequent editorials (pieces characterized by one medical historian as "comfortably free of logic") would have been well known among physicians in Illinois. Whalen had served as president of both the Chicago Medical Society and the ISMS before taking charge of the journal in 1919, a post he retained undisputedly until his death in 1941.[55]

The bitter debate over Sheppard-Towner in Illinois was all the more remarkable for its distinctly gendered dimension. Condemnations of the growing power of the federal government frequently emphasized the fact that these unwelcome, meddlesome Washington bureaucrats were women. Some Sheppard-Towner opponents argued that placing maternal and child health programs under the auspices of the female-dominated Children's Bureau represented mere appeals to "sentimentality" rather than the promotion of sound and responsible social policy. Highlighting the fact that many administrators in the Children's Bureau had never married, some commentators suggested that these women (whom the inimitable Whalen disparaged as "derailed menopausics") were really motivated in their work on behalf of the nation's children by their own unfulfilled maternal instincts. Other Sheppard-Towner opponents saw an even more ominous sign in the growing female political influence in Washington. A favorite theme of Whalen's editorials in the *Illinois Medical Journal* alleged that the women of the Children's Bureau had developed close ties to the Soviets and were secretly engaged in an international conspiracy to take over the United States. One piece cited as "proof" the distribution of a pamphlet entitled "Maternity Benefit Systems in Foreign Countries," which Whalen claimed to be "socialistic and bolshevistic in almost every line." Whalen, however, apparently had confused the Children's Bureau with the Women's Bureau, recently organized within the U.S. Department of Labor, which had actually published the pamphlet he cited.[56]

By the 1920s, then, the ideology of maternalism as a force for social reform had lost much of its potency; the formerly undisputed place women held in health and social welfare advocacy during the Progressive Era had now become contested ground. Following close upon the heels of the maternalist victory the Sheppard-Towner Act represented, a severe backlash ensued against women holding positions of power, a reaction aimed particularly at officials in the Children's Bureau. Further, as historian Molly Ladd-Taylor has observed, the intensity of this backlash seems in retrospect to have been strangely out of proportion to the relative modesty of the provisions and budget of the act itself. A closer look, however, reveals that the distinctly gendered dimension to the contest over Sheppard-Towner — a feature clearly notable in the heated Illinois debate — reflected an even deeper controversy concerning the delineation of power boundaries in the evolving welfare state.[57]

In addition to officials in the Children's Bureau, Whalen and his anti-Sheppard-Towner allies in Illinois also assailed the women lobbyists who had recently converged on the state capital urging their representatives to vote in favor of enabling legislation. Female supporters of the Sheppard-Towner Act were portrayed by turns as avaricious, unpatriotic, devious, dangerous, or just plain pushy. The ILWV's lobbying tactic of interviewing legislators and recording their views on index cards presented an especially disturbing sight. One editorial asked whether the citizens of Illinois were willing to stand by passively as these unnaturally aggressive "Meddlesome Matties" intruded into the "past histories and private affairs of every home, [just] as these women have card-indexed legislators to intimidate them into enacting such bills as the Sheppard-Towner bill."[58] The spectacle of women lobbyists eagerly jumping into the fray of Illinois state politics — and apparently holding their own — undoubtedly startled many observers of the capital scene.

The role of female nurses, as opposed to male doctors, within the maternal and child health programs proposed under Sheppard-Towner came under attack as well. A number of physicians strongly objected to Dr. Rawlings's plan to give nurses supervisory authority within health education programs, asserting that preventive health work must remain the exclusive domain of medical doctors. Although they did receive formal medical training and were licensed by the state, public health nurses were unqualified, in ISMS president Charles Humiston's view, to provide instruction on health matters. "I do not recognize the so-called nursing profession as a profession pure and simple," he asserted during his testimony to the House committee. "But nurses are *assistants* to the medical practice in its proper and wide sense. They are carrying out orders, and if you permit nurses to act on their own initiative, then they are practicing medicine, which is in conflict with the laws of every state."[59] But, in their denunciations, physicians occasionally took aim at nurses precisely because they were women. In March 1923, the *Illinois Medical Journal* forecasted that, should enabling legislation be passed in the state, "It will be a great day for the traveling nurse who can talk to her tongue's content, telling women how to take care of themselves during their maternity period." These nurses, Whalen continued, would not work under the supervision of physicians but instead under the "undisputed despotism of the chief of the Children's Bureau." A later editorial predicted that "at the present rate of socialistic legislation . . . the medical profession will have been legislated out of existence and surpassed in its entirety by the overtrained and — say it softly — over ignorant nurse."[60] Understandably, such highly charged and gratuitously vindictive rhetoric had a chilling effect on public health nurses themselves. Nurses were placed into the extremely uncomfortable position of incurring the wrath of the powerful state medical society if they came out publicly in support of legislation that would unquestionably benefit their own professional development. Mabel M. Dunlap, president of the Illinois State Association of Graduate Nurses, wrote to the ILWV to say that, because of her organization's "peculiar relationship with the medical profession, I must ask that our Association be omitted from the list of those endorsing the Bill." Dunlap made this request despite her own "hearty sympathy" for Sheppard-Towner, adding, "I think you will understand the situation as it affects our Association."[61] Under such gendered professional attacks, Illinois public health nurses found their voices effectively silenced during the Sheppard-Towner debate.

By the time the Illinois General Assembly voted on enabling legislation, thirty-nine states had already adopted the Sheppard-Towner Act's provisions. (The legislatures of Delaware, Minnesota, New Hampshire, and New Mexico, in fact, had voted to accept the act even before its final passage in Washington.)[62] The bill was introduced into the Illinois House on March 7, 1923, and subsequently referred to the Committee on Appropriations. The identical Senate bill was introduced on March 13, 1923, and referred to the Committee on Public Health, Hygiene, and Sanitation. In debating the bill in the Senate Committee, legislators reprised the by now familiar themes citing the potential dangers of government paternalism and the need for more fiscal responsibility. Senator Charles Dunlap of Champaign County, responding to charges that too much paternalism already existed in the state's programs for bovine tuberculosis control, road improvement, and agricultural extension work, remarked that "whatever our ideas may be about paternalism . . . it is mighty poor to begin [cutting back] on infants and mothers." (Senator Dunlap was the husband of Nora Dunlap, the energetic supporter of maternal and child health education activities in the Illinois Farmers' Institute.) Senator Kessinger of Kane County concurred: "I would like to kill Federal aid, but I am going to try and kill it some other day in some other way. I vote 'aye.'" Mr. Swift of Lake County presented the pragmatic argument that "for the two years that are left of the Sheppard-Towner Act I vote that we take our part of the Federal money." When Senator Webster of Cook County objected to the idea of "sending people that have never had any children into the homes to interfere with and tell the mothers how to raise children," Senator Glenn of Jackson County had a ready reply: "You might as well say that you wouldn't employ a physician or specialist at Mayo's to operate upon you for appendicitis or for concussion of the brain simply because he had never been operated upon himself for appendicitis or concussion of the brain." Senator Barbour of Cook County expressed his resentment of the heavy-handed lobbying tactics used by anti-Sheppard-Towner physicians in his district: "They seem to think they own me." Senator Barbour's remark was duly reported in the pages of the *Illinois Medical Journal*, and the editor slyly urged doctors to take note of their own state senators' public remarks about the medical profession, promising that "the data will be found useful at some subsequent date." On May 22, 1923, the Senate Committee recommended the bill's passage by a vote of twenty-seven to eight. The bill, however, eventually met its demise in the Committee on Appropriations, which over the next several weeks steadfastly refused to fund it. By this time, the state's fiscal clock had run out, and as a consequence the identical House bill died as well. Enabling legislation had not survived its ordeal in the Illinois General Assembly.[63]

Clearly disappointed, the ILWV nevertheless hoped to reintroduce enabling legislation when the General Assembly met again in 1925. At this point, however, Isaac Rawlings had become extremely pessimistic about the fate of public health legislation in the state capital. The rancorous disputes that had characterized recent political struggles over public health provision in the state had proven difficult for the embattled director of the ISDPH. The most recent sparring over Sheppard-Towner only served to convince Rawlings that "physicians in the state were rabid against state medicine." Any new public health initiatives must now be undertaken with the utmost care and delicacy. Although he was the designated administrator of Sheppard-Towner programs in Illinois, Rawlings apparently was no longer willing to actively defy his powerful physician colleagues in the ISMS after the turmoil of 1923. He advised Caroline McCready of the ILWV that any future plans to reintroduce federally sponsored maternal and infant health programs in Illinois would have to be "approached with a scientific and persuasive attitude, those working for this education forgetting the heat of argument and ugly spirit which has pervaded all groups who have been for or against the acceptance of the Sheppard-Towner Act."[64]

By contrast, the ISMS was heartened by the success of its efforts to defeat enabling legislation in the Illinois General Assembly, sustaining its vigorous opposition to federally sponsored maternal and child health education programs over the next four years. As late as 1927, one analyst of federal health policy pointed to persistent opposition from the ISMS as the cause of

Illinois' continued "aloofness" from the Sheppard-Towner Act. The influential national reform journal, *The Survey*, found the state's refusal to cooperate with Sheppard-Towner difficult to explain, for as one editorial comment put it, Illinois could hardly be "distinguished by brilliant progress in reducing its infant death rate."[65] With Rawlings's loss of political nerve, however, the fate of enabling legislation in Illinois had apparently been sealed. In helping to keep the opposition alive, the ISMS played a key role in the Sheppard-Towner Act's eventual demise at the national level as well.

By the time the act came up for renewal in Congress in 1926 organized medicine, led by the burgeoning AMA, had gained considerable political clout and the national-level opposition was now much more forceful than it had been in 1921. AMA leaders also had learned something about mounting a war of words from organized physicians in Illinois, and the *Journal of the American Medical Association*, like the *Illinois Medical Journal*, now editorialized at length concerning the iniquities of Sheppard-Towner. After a congressional brawl and a filibuster led by the act's opponents, the parties reached a compromise in which the law was renewed for a period of two years only. In 1929 the Sheppard-Towner Act was repealed.[66]

Throughout the remainder of the 1920s Illinois public health advocates and their maternalist allies continued to face enormous difficulties in translating their ideals and goals into politically viable realities. Historian Thomas R. Pegram notes that an extremely diverse array of rival interest groups, each with its own fiercely loyal constituency, fought for control of Illinois politics in this period. Newly enfranchised women in the state, despite their impressive experience in grassroots organizing, found themselves virtually shut out of entrenched male political machines in the years following the suffrage victory.[67] Progressive health reformers had entered the political arena convinced that an inherent public interest lay in improving the health of women and children in their state. Their strategy had rested — perhaps rather naively — on the faith that, once the citizens of Illinois clearly understood the public benefits to be derived from federally sponsored maternal and child health programs, they would join forces to rally in support of bringing Sheppard-Towner to their state. But, while "baby-saving" carried a wide public appeal throughout Illinois, this grassroots popularity did not automatically translate into mass political support for the expansion of the welfare state.

Unlike the prewar preventive health campaigns, enabling legislation for Sheppard-Towner did not play out as an intrinsic public good helping to bring modernity to the state, but rather as one special interest counted among many — all competing for patronage in the General Assembly. The political corruption running rampant in Illinois in the 1920s undoubtedly added to the difficulties faced by health reformers new to that state's political scene. Historians have characterized the tenure of Governor Len Small (1920–1928), in fact, as unparalleled in mismanagement, fraud, intrigue, and "downright disregard of the public interest." Small's lack of reticence about appropriating public funds resulted in an indictment and fines of over one million dollars. Meanwhile in Chicago, Health Commissioner Herman Bundesen was forced to resign his post in 1927 when he refused to insert campaign literature from Mayor "Big Bill" Thompson into a Chicago Board of Health pamphlet on baby care.[68] Political support for maternal and child health programs in Illinois, it seems, came with some disagreeable strings attached.

Lacking political clout, supporters of Sheppard-Towner in Illinois faced an immense challenge from a powerful business-medical alliance that defined the best interest of the public to be in limiting the scope of state and federal government intrusion into health care provision. The Sheppard-Towner Act represented yet another perceived threat to the integrity of private enterprise, including private medical practice in Illinois. When faced with a such a direct and heavy-handed political challenge from his colleagues in the ISMS, the beleaguered chief of that state's public health bureaucracy had blinked, thereby surrendering an unparalleled opportunity to reap what years of health reform activism had sown.

For its part, the ISMS continued to contest virtually any attempt to enlarge the scope of public health activities, denouncing all state-sponsored health activities in Illinois as inherent threats to private medical interests. In 1924 for example, following the rancorous debate over Sheppard-Towner the previous year, the ISDPH was forced to shut down its diagnostic clinics for polio victims due to "some unfavorable feeling in the ranks of the medical profession." Physicians had raised objections that diagnostic activities such as giving "advice as to shoes, casts, and braces" to polio victims crossed the line into the actual medical treatment of these patients.[69] Even the venerable Infant Welfare Society of Chicago, a private philanthropy that since 1911 had used the volunteer services of scores of doctors and nurses in infant health work among Chicago's immigrant communities, came under attack in a series of letters to the editor of the *Illinois Medical Journal* in 1927. Under a headline proclaiming that the "Infant Welfare Society is Practicing Medicine," Emmet Keating of the ISMS charged that the Society was "trying to overcome [maternal ignorance] by educating mothers to keep away from their neighborhood physicians and giving the impression that the physicians employed by the Infant Welfare Society are highly competent." By the end of the decade, organized physicians in Illinois had developed an unshakable conviction that the interests of private medical practice and public health efforts were irreconcilable.[70]

If preventive health care practices moved increasingly into the realm of the private consumption of goods and services in Illinois, however, it is also clear that *access* to these things did not necessarily become any easier, especially for the poorest and most remote residents of the state. Medical historians have described the declining fortunes of both public health nursing services and the neighborhood health dispensary in this period, along with the simultaneous rise of the hospital as the primary American health care institution. But not everyone, of course, could avail themselves of these new institutions. By the mid-1920s, for example, medical services at Provident Hospital had severely deteriorated under exorbitant pressures to meet virtually all of the health care needs of Chicago's black population, which had burgeoned during the First World War. The availability of health care services for African Americans simply could not keep pace with their numbers migrating into the city, and as late as 1946, a U.S. Public Health Service report indicated that the racial health care gap had not been significantly reduced.[71]

The dwindling number of country physicians was also an issue of considerable concern to farm women. "Where's the doctor when you need him?" the popular rural women's magazine, *The Farmer's Wife*, demanded to know in 1928. "The number of rural doctors is rapidly growing less, the distance between farm homes and doctors' offices is becoming greater, and the cost of medical service is getting higher." A study published the following year estimated that public health services were available to less than 20 percent of American farm families.[72] While the rural population of Illinois did become less numerous during the period under study here, the proportion of physicians practicing in small towns and rural areas also decreased noticeably. Census figures show that, while in 1910 48 percent of the state's physicians practiced in towns of less than 25,000, by 1930 this proportion had shrunk to just 30 percent. (Conversely, the proportion practicing in Chicago alone grew from 43 percent in 1910 to 54 percent in 1930.)[73]

A 1930 investigation of public health conditions in Illinois found that, while Chicago's stillbirth rate had declined by 7 percent during the 1920s, the rate for rural areas had actually *increased* by 4.1 percent. These examiners theorized that differences in the availability of prenatal care between

Chicago and rural downstate residents may have been the key.[74] The health care services gap between rural and urban dwellers, including those in Illinois, would only become wider during the Great Depression. Even though country dwellers composed 26.4 percent of the population of Illinois in 1940, only 13 percent of the state's physicians practiced in rural areas. A contemporary study calculated that only one physician was available for every 1,730 rural residents of Illinois.[75]

Bringing modernity to Illinois remained a viable aspiration in this period, and concern for the health of the women and children of Illinois did not die out with the defeat of enabling legislation for the Sheppard-Towner Act in 1923. Many of the preventive health education activities that had preceded the Sheppard-Towner debate — including better baby contests and Home Bureau demonstrations of the latest methods of household sanitation — continued unabated without the aid of federal funding. Such activities did not pose a political problem for health reformers, however, because they reinforced rather than challenged the privatized, medicalized model of modernity that physicians and business leaders supported — social progress through the consumption of goods and services. One important purpose of the ever-popular better baby contests, for example, was to encourage mothers to utilize the services of local medical professionals in caring for their own and their children's health.

The shift away from a more socially conscious approach to health reform and toward a model stressing the private consumption of health care services may be seen clearly in the formation of a new State Advisory Committee on Child Hygiene in 1925. The new committee included representatives of both the ISMS and the ISDPH along with the Illinois State Dental Society, the Illinois Federation of Women's Clubs, and the Illinois Council of the Parent-Teacher Association. Although nonmedical agencies were represented, the scope of activities to be undertaken by the new committee was notably more circumscribed than the broadly conceived and socially ambitious aims that had distinguished Progressive Era health reform efforts in Illinois. The function of the State Advisory Committee apparently consisted solely of ensuring publicity for "the special programs and campaigns undertaken by state health officials."[76] The specter of enlisting the federal government in aid of preventive health care education programs for mothers and children in Illinois would not be raised again.

EPILOGUE

The extraordinary imagination and drive with which preventive health reformers carried out their campaigns for modernity in the early twentieth century remains palpable in the historical evidence they left behind. Even today one is tempted to become caught up in the sheer excitement they created, and in doing so it would be all too easy to pronounce their ambitious efforts to produce a healthier citizenry an unqualified success. But, because a number of variables changed simultaneously in the years between 1900 and 1930, the job of evaluating the results of health reform constitutes something of a Promethean task. While demographic evidence demonstrates that a major transition to both lower mortality rates and increased life expectancy did occur sometime around 1900, identifying precise cause-and-effect relationships within this shift is an exercise fraught with peril. Historian Richard A. Meckel recently has argued that a definitive pronouncement on the success of the Progressive Era infant welfare movement would be premature at present because too many key variables are still unknown including ethnic, racial, and regional differences in mortality and morbidity. Taking into account all of the environmental conditions influencing specific causes of death in young children further complicates the attempt at historical analysis. Likewise, scholars endeavoring to explain the reductions in maternal mortality which became evident after the 1930s have concluded that progress most likely resulted not from a single cause but rather from a combination of factors such as the development of antibiotics and sulfonamides, better obstetrical training for medical professionals, and improved public awareness and open discussion of issues concerning pregnancy and childbirth.[1]

Nevertheless, if we cannot with complete confidence draw a straight line connecting preventive health and hygiene campaigns to the lower

Table 6.1
Trend in Illinois Infant Mortality, 1910–1930

Year	Rate[a]
1910	149.9
1916	119.9[b]
1920	87.5
1925	72.5
1930	55.8

Sources: Illinois State Planning Commission, *Infant Mortality in Illinois* (1934); Rawlings, *The Rise and Fall of Disease in Illinois* (1927): 394.

[a]Deaths of infants under one year of age, per 1,000 live births.

[b]Data for 1915 were not available.

mortality rates realized in these years, this much at least seems certain: Because protection against contagion represented the most powerful weapon available for combatting illness and disease in the early twentieth century, popular campaigns promoting basic prophylactic measures such as hand washing, boiling well water before drinking it, and feeding babies pasteurized milk in sterilized bottles represented a critical means for improving the life chances of individuals. Before the availability of infection-fighting drugs, the widespread adoption of more hygienic practices by thousands of mothers within their own homes saved a significant number of children's lives. Nor should we overlook the fact that better attention to matters of personal, domestic, and community hygiene undoubtedly improved the overall quality of life for many urban and rural dwellers alike.

Changes in America's heartland reflected the national demographic trends. Although maternal death rates in Illinois remained relatively high until the later 1930s, that state did witness a dramatic overall decrease in infant mortality, from 140 per 1,000 live births in 1907 to just under 56 in 1930 (table 6.1.). In 1934, an Illinois state planning commission reported with evident satisfaction that for the first time ever that state's infant death rate (52.8) had fallen below the national figure (59.9).[2] Keeping in mind that larger social, political, and economic changes in Illinois undoubtedly influenced these outcomes to varying degrees as well, the contributions made by institutional policymakers, public health practitioners, maternalist social welfare activists, and agricultural extension agents in realizing such success nevertheless must be acknowledged.

As this study has demonstrated, mothers themselves were no less significant in bringing about such a historically significant transition in Illinois. Health reformers placed women at the very center of their efforts, assigning mothers the urgent imperative to educate themselves about the latest preventive health and hygiene methods and then to put this information to good use in improving their own homes, neighborhoods, and communities. Rural and urban women made progress happen when they carried their little ones to neighborhood pure milk stations, listened attentively to household hygiene demonstrations, scrutinized mechanical exhibits at community public health fairs, and watched with hopeful anticipation as baby contest judges weighed and measured their children at the Illinois state fair. With crucial support from volunteer women activists, the message of modernization through preventive health and hygiene was carried to cities, towns, and rural areas throughout the state. Mothers' responses, in turn, both shaped the specific contours of hundreds of local health reform campaigns and contributed significantly to the movement's overall momentum over the course of three decades.

But any attempt to evaluate the effectiveness of preventive health reform campaigns must deal with their deficiencies as well as their successes, for such efforts took place within a distinct set of limitations. Rigid racial barriers segregated black and white public health movements in Chicago, for example, while cultural misunderstandings and tensions pervaded health reform activities taking place in that city's immigrant neighborhoods. Although agrarian uplifters ostensibly included all mothers in their persistent call to bring modernity to rural Illinois, it was only relatively affluent farm women who found themselves in a position to respond. Socioeconomic differences between the state's northern and southern regions — a characteristic clearly evident in the social landscape of Illinois since the mid-nineteenth century — grew even more pronounced over the course of the 1920s.

Despite experiencing a "golden age" of agriculture, deep pockets of rural poverty persisted in Illinois. The steady process of farm closures that had alarmed agrarian uplifters before the First World War accelerated dramatically with the collapse of the agricultural economy by the end of the decade. By 1930, farmland in Lake County, located north of Cook County along Lake Michigan, was valued at $329 per acre while land in Pope County, at the extreme southern end of the state, stood at only $21 per acre.[3] Interestingly, variations in the incidence of public health problems among Illinois residents, including rates of infant mortality, tuberculosis, and typhoid fever, followed this distinctive north-south pattern.

Grouping counties together by region in 1927, Illinois public health officials found that the 33 northernmost counties experienced a combined infant mortality rate of 65.7, while the rate for the 35 counties representing the state's central region came in at 67.4. In striking contrast, the 34 southernmost counties in Illinois had a combined infant mortality rate of 88.2. Cairo, in southernmost Alexander County, stood out among Illinois cities with over 115 infant deaths per 1,000 births, while Chicago's rate was recorded as just 66.56. (Unfortunately, Cairo's public health problems had persisted since Charles Dickens had first chronicled his displeasure with that city in 1842.) In addition, this 1927 study by the Illinois State Department of Public Health commented on the fact that infant mortality rates remained markedly higher in rural areas than in cities containing a population of 10,000 or more.[4] If Illinois was well on its way to reaching modernity through the production of a healthier populace, such progress lay along a decidedly uneven path.

Although work still remained to be done in that state's health reform movement, the larger context within which preventive health and hygiene campaigns operated had clearly changed. In their insistence that better health for all the state's residents constituted an inherent public good as well as a desirable private benefit, reformers carried preventive health care from within the confines of the individual household and into the public arena — where it became exposed to a level of discord and debate unanticipated by reformers themselves. The unprecedented attention to health care's wider social meanings engendered by wartime baby-saving crusades raised new and difficult questions about where the ultimate responsibility for a healthier populace lay. Sharp differences between partisans of public and private health services erupted full-blown after the First World War when the unprecedented role of government in safeguarding maternal and child health became the subject of a rancorous political debate. In 1923, Illinois maternalists' failure to secure their state's participation in the Sheppard-Towner Act marked a critical transition toward the more medicalized and privatized orientation in preventive health care that took place during the 1920s.

This shift in the ideological underpinnings of preventive health care went hand-in-hand with a discernible subsiding of maternalism as a source of women's public power. Thus, while the Progressive Era's overriding goal of lower infant mortality rates was in fact realized in the 1920s, such progress came in the absence of an accompanying discourse empowering mothers as special agents of modernity. Instead, as the residents of Illinois steadily became a less rural and more urban people, women's role as consumers within the modern private household took on a new and unrivaled importance. The higher health standards so successfully promulgated by progressive reformers had prompted a virtual explosion in consumer products ostensibly meant to help mothers attain them. Throughout the decade ubiquitous magazine, newspaper, and radio advertisements exhorted "Mrs. Consumer" to safeguard her family's well-being by purchasing everything from Lysol disinfectant to bottled vitamins to prepackaged foods. Historians of advertising have noted the intense concerns about personal hygiene and household cleanliness that seemed to hang like a free-floating anxiety around the pages of popular magazines in this period, especially those aimed at a readership of middle-class women. Soap manufacturers allied in the "Cleanliness Institute," for example, marketed their personal and household cleaning products as health aids in advertisements that featured women and children prominently, reminding their readers that family health and well-being depended upon a mother's ability to choose her purchases wisely. At the same time, pharmaceutical companies plugging newly available nutritional supplements exploited women's fears that their perfectly healthy-seeming children could actually be suffering from debilitating vitamin deficiencies. Meanwhile the burgeoning field of home economics, which had provided vital institutional support for preventive health reform campaigns in Illinois, underwent a sea change of its own in this period. Once leading the way in promoting higher education and a pivotal role for women in the public sphere, home economists increasingly concentrated their attentions on grooming women to become modern consumers of goods and services.[5] Captured by private enterprise, the movement to promote preventive health and hygiene now lacked a vigorous maternalist voice expounding the wider public mission of mothers' work in health care.

If better health were indeed purchasable by the modern mother trained in consumer economics, then the general public had no real cause for concern that preventable disease and untimely death persisted among particular populations. Ironically, Progressive Era reformers' argument that a higher standard of health lay within a mother's control actually made it considerably easier to ignore any remaining disparities in infant mortality rates within the state. In an age enlightened by the germ theory and advanced hygiene education it had also become more politically viable to blame the persistence of poor health on the willful negligence of mothers themselves, ignoring conditions such as grinding poverty, poorly constructed and unsanitary housing, or lack of access to either public or private medical care — factors affecting health which remained largely beyond an individual woman's ability to control. Clean homes, healthy children, and orderly communities, of course, had lost none of their potency as symbols of middle-class respectability in 1930, and in an age of sophisticated mass advertising such dreams actually seemed more attainable than ever before. Although it remained a powerful signifier of upward mobility in America's heartland, modern motherhood no longer represented the vital foundation of wide-ranging social change.

NOTES

Introduction

1. The epigraph is from Hedger's presentation.

2. Tomes, *Gospel of Germs*, pp. 157–59.

3. On the relationship between social welfare and public health reform activism in the United States during the early twentieth century, see the following works: Fee, *Disease and Discovery*; Leavitt, *Typhoid Mary* and *The Healthiest City*; Meckel, *Save the Babies*; Rogers, *Dirt and Disease*; Rosen, *Preventive Medicine*; Rosenkrantz, *Public Health and the State*; Starr, *Social Transformation*. Historians' efforts to reach a consensus on defining the "Progressive Era" are reviewed in Rodgers, "In Search of Progressivism."

4. Meckel, *Save the Babies*, pp. 103–9, 159.

5. Duffy, *The Sanitarians*, p. 207; Rosen, *Preventive Health*, pp. 20–35; Starr, *Social Transformation*, pp. 189–94.

6. Starr, *Social Transformation*, p. 32. On gender and nineteenth-century health reforms, see Fee and Greene, "Women and Public Health"; Hoy, *Chasing Dirt*; Morantz, "Making Women Modern"; Numbers, "Do-It-Yourself the Sectarian Way"; Tomes, "The Private Side of Public Health."

7. Infant Welfare Society of Chicago, *Infant Welfare Society of Chicago, Annual Report*, 1915. Infant Welfare Society of Chicago, records, Box 3, folder 2-3. On "scientific motherhood," see Apple, *Mothers and Medicine*, pp. 97–113; Ladd-Taylor, *Mother-Work*, p. 4.

8. The historiography of women, gender, and the American welfare state is growing in volume as well as in depth. Recent examples include Gordon, ed., *Women, the State, and Welfare*; Gordon, *Pitied But Not Entitled*; Klaus, *Every Child a Lion*; Seth Koven and Sonya Michel, eds., *Mothers of a New World*; Ladd-Taylor, *Raising a Baby the Government Way* and *Mother-Work*; Michel and Rosen, "The Paradox of Maternalism"; Muncy, *Creating a Female Dominion*; Rothman, "Women's Clinics or Doctors' Offices?"; Schackel, *Social Housekeepers*; Sklar, *Florence Kelley*; Skocpol, *Protecting Soldiers and Mothers*.

9. Klaus, *Every Child a Lion*, p. 137; Bonner, *Medicine in Chicago, 1850–1950*, pp. 175–98; Rawlings, *Rise and Fall*, pp. 127–35.

10. Frank and Jerome, eds., *Annals of the Chicago Woman's Club*, p. 21.

11. Hart, *Pleasure Is Mine*, pp. 200–201; Bonner, *Medicine in Chicago*, p. 156; Muncy, *Creating a Female Dominion*, pp. 47–51.

12. See, for example, Skocpol, *Protecting Soldiers and Mothers*, pp. 1–66.

13. Bonner, *Medicine in Chicago*, pp. 186–92; Haas, *152 Years of Municipal Health Care*, pp. 7–8.

14. Rogers, *Dirt and Disease*, p. 7; Hoy, *Chasing Dirt*, p. 88.

15. Neth, *Preserving the Family Farm*, pp. 98–99, 123.

16. My interpretation of health reformers' attitudes in Illinois is consistent with Alan Kraut's view that those who worked in public health were ethnocentric but rarely virulently nativistic. Kraut, *Silent Travelers*, p. 134. Historian Linda Gordon has pointed out that progressive social welfare activists manifested so much concern with acculturating immigrants precisely because they believed them to be "salvageable." Gordon, *Pitied But Not Entitled*, pp. 84–85. Alisa Klaus distinguishes the environmental rationale used by maternal and child health reformers in the United States from the more overtly eugenicist arguments put forward by their contemporaries in France. Klaus, "Depopulation and Race Suicide," pp. 188–210.

17. Historian Alisa Klaus has argued that activists in the Children's Bureau interpreted the persistence of high rates of maternal mortality as evidence of the oppression of women. Klaus, *Every Child a Lion*, p. 230.

18. Cowan and Cowan, *Our Parents' Lives*, p. 143.

19. Works privileging a clients' perspective on Progressive Era reform include Gordon, *Heroes of Their Own Lives*; Stadum, *Poor Women and Their Families*; and Schackel, *Social Housekeepers*.

20. "Women and Their Duties," *Dziennik Zwiazkowy* (February 4, 1908). Chicago Foreign Language Press Survey.

21. Smith, "'Sick and Tired,'" pp. 1–56; Hine, *Black Women in White*, p. 31.

22. Bonner, *Medicine in Chicago*, pp. 7, 176–77, 181–92; Rawlings, "Rise and Fall," p. 304; Davenport, "Sanitation Revolution," pp. 309–10; Haas, *152 Years of Municipal Health Care*, pp. 7–8.

23. Midwestern farmers, including those in Illinois, were overwhelmingly white and native-born in this period. For a discussion of the racial and ethnic composition of midwestern farmers, see Jellison, *Entitled to Power*, pp. 5–10.

24. Lentzner, "Seasonal Patterns," p. 15; Bonner, *Medicine in Chicago*, p. 7; Rawlings, *Rise and Fall*, p. 35.

25. Fulmer, "Rural Nursing Service in Cook County," p. 59.

26. *Report of the Health Insurance Commission of the State of Illinois, May 1, 1919*, p. 7.

27. On the Country Life Movement, see Bowers, *The Country Life Movement in America*; Danbom, *The Resisted Revolution*; Kirschner, *City and Country*; Jellison, *Entitled to Power*; Neth, *Preserving the Family Farm*.

28. Ironically, this delayed attention to rural areas is paralleled by historical scholarship today as the distinctive ways in which public health and social welfare

campaigns developed outside of major industrial cities remain largely unexamined. Richard A. Meckel has challenged historians of health care to investigate areas outside of large cities in "Judging Progressive Era Infant Welfare," pp. 109–10.

29. Rothman, "Women's Clinics or Doctors' Offices?" p. 188.

30. "Infant Welfare Society Practicing Medicine," p. 279.

Chapter 1

1. Hedger, "Report of the Campaign Against Summer Diarrhea," pp. 534–47; Chicago Community Trust, *Prenatal Care in Chicago*, p. 26.

2. Bonner, *Medicine in Chicago*, p. 29; Lentzner, "Seasonal Patterns," pp. 19–22. Lentzner points out that, while such apparent differentials may be due to variations in statistical reporting among the various cities, these proportions nevertheless do reflect extremely high infant mortality rates in Chicago, especially by present-day standards.

3. Lentzner, "Seasonal Patterns," pp. 26–32; Bonner, *Medicine in Chicago*, p. 30.

4. *Report of the Health Insurance Commission of the State of Illinois* (Springfield, 1919), p. 68; Chicago Department of Public Health, *Report for 1911–1918* (Chicago, 1919); Chicago Community Trust, *Prenatal Care in Chicago*, p. 26.

5. Hoffert, *Private Matters*, p. 149.

6. Bonner, *Medicine in Chicago*, pp. 186–92; Davenport, "Sanitation Revolution," p. 310; Haas, *152 Years of Municipal Health Care*, pp. 7–8. On nineteenth-century sanitarianism, see Duffy, *The Sanitarians*; Rosen, *Preventive Medicine in the United States*; Starr, *The Social Transformation of American Medicine*.

7. Bonner, *Medicine in Chicago*, pp. 61–62; Hart, *Pleasure Is Mine*, pp. 200–201; "Hedger, Caroline (Miss)," *Who's Who in Chicago* (1926), p. 399; McCarthy, *Noblesse Oblige*, pp. 154–55. On the close connections between middle-class women and female physicians in the nineteenth century, see Drachman, "Female Solidarity and Professional Success" and Fee and Greene, "Science and Social Reform."

8. Burgess, "This Beautiful Charity," p. 51. On district nursing in London, see Ross, *Love and Toil*; Hoy, *Chasing Dirt*, pp. 76–78.

9. Hedger, "Report of the Campaign Against Summer Diarrhea," p. 536; "Elizabeth McCormick Memorial Fund," pamphlet, 1912. Records of the Elizabeth McCormick Memorial Fund, folder 193; "Mrs. Harriet Hammond McCormick" (obituary). *Woman's City Club Bulletin* 9 (February 1921): p. 9.

10. *Woman's City Club Bulletin* 8 (January 1920): p. 8; Infant Welfare Society of Chicago, "The First Ten Years of the Woman's Auxiliary of the Infant Welfare Society of Chicago," Infant Welfare Society of Chicago, records, Box 1, folder 1-1.

11. Antler and Fox, "The Movement Toward a Safe Maternity," pp. 490–505; Klaus, "Women's Organizations and the Infant Health Movement," p. 157; Klaus, *Every Child a Lion*, p. 170; Litoff, *American Midwife Debate*, p. 28; Muncy, *Creating a Female Dominion*, pp. xiii–xiv; Wertz and Wertz, *Lying-In*, p. 155.

12. Farnham, *Life in Prairie Land*, pp. 49–56.

13. Bonner, *Medicine in Chicago*, pp. 23–31.

14. *Annual Report of the Illinois State Board of Health*; Chicago Department of Health, *Mortality Statistics, 1912–1918*, p. 1234; Chicago Community Trust, *Prenatal Care in Chicago*, pp. 20–45; Reagan, *When Abortion Was a Crime*, pp. 76–79.

15. A description of prenatal services in neighborhood dispensaries may be found in the Chicago Community Trust's 1922 report, *Prenatal Care in Chicago*, pp. 41–47.

16. Hamilton, "Excessive Child-Bearing," p. 183.

17. Hoy, *Chasing Dirt*, pp. 96–97; Hedger, "The Unhealthfulness of Packingtown," pp. 7507–10; Breckinridge and Abbott, "Housing Conditions in Chicago," pp. 433–68.

18. McDowell, Mary, papers, "Standard of Living: Civic Frontiersmen," typescript, 1914 [?], folder 13.

19. Interview #BLA-144. Oral History Archives of Chicago Polonia.

20. McDowell, papers, "The Immigrant American," unnumbered typescript, folder 12; Barrett, *Work and Community*, p. 69.

21. McDowell, papers, Caroline Hedger, "Health: Summer, 1908," typescript, folder 13.

22. Loudon, "Maternal Mortality," p. 199; Chicago Department of Public Health, *Mortality Statistics, 1912–1918*, p. 1234; Chicago Community Trust, *Prenatal Care in Chicago*, pp. 20–45.

23. Rosen, *Preventive Medicine in the United States*, pp. 27–32.

24. F. S. Churchill, "Studies in Chicago Philanthropy" (1913). Infant Welfare Society of Chicago, Box 2, folder 2-2; "Minutes of the Milk Commission June 11, 1903." Infant Welfare Society of Chicago, Box 1, folder 1-7; Lentzner, "Seasonal Patterns," pp. 299–301. On the politics of dairy reform in Illinois, see Pegram, "Public Health and Progressive Dairying in Illinois," pp. 36–60.

25. Dickens, *American Notes*, pp. 197–98.

26. Medical Officers' Journals, Box 1, folder 3a (January 24, 1880–July 1, 1897), United States Marine Hospital Service (Cairo, Illinois), records; Gates, *Illinois Central Railroad*, p. 238.

27. *Cairo Weekly Times* (January 9, 1856) quoted in Jane Adams, *Transformation of Rural Life*, p. 257 n. 3.

28. Carlson, "Black Migration," pp. 37–46; Smukstra, "Work and Family," pp. 35–56, 48–81.

29. "Outpatient Register, March 1911–December 1914," Box 14, folder 1, United States Marine Hospital Service (Cairo, Illinois), records; Kirschner, *City and Country*, p. 13; Rosen, *Preventive Medicine*, p. 20; Leavitt, *Typhoid Mary*, pp. 14–58; Miller and Montgomery, *A Chautauqua to Remember*, pp. 158–64.

30. "Typhoid Fever at Tuscola," p. 143; "Problems of the Smaller Illinois Community," p. 115.; "New Contagious Disease Cards," p. 196.

31. McAdam, "National Menace," p. 322. Census data are cited in Jellison, *Entitled to Power*, p. 55.

32. Bartow, *Chemical and Biological Survey of the Waters of Illinois*, p. 79.

33. Bevier, Isabel, papers, "Address, January, 1917, Resume of the Report of the Farm Home Survey by Charles L. Stewart"; Nauss, "Typhoid Fever at Tuscola," p. 279.

34. Meigs, "Rural Obstetrics," pp. 61–75. Dorothy Reed Mendenhall's comments on the failure to record puerperal septicemia as a cause of death are found in the discussion following Meigs's presentation.

35. Bartow, *Chemical and Biological Survey of the Waters of Illinois*, p. 79; Lentzer, "Seasonal Patterns," p. 345.

36. Rawlings, *Rise and Fall*, pp. 202, 300. For a discussion of the political battle over milk regulation in Illinois, see Pegram, "Public Health and Progressive Dairying in Illinois," pp. 36–50.

37. Bonner, *Medicine in Chicago*, p. 137; "Fulmer, Harriet (Miss)," Marquis, ed., *Book of Chicagoans*, p. 251.

38. Foster and Fulmer, "Health Survey," pp. 30–32.

39. Foster and Fulmer, "Health Survey," pp. 30–33. Historian James Harvey Young has estimated that in the early twentieth century, Americans spent over $74 million annually on patent medicines. *Medical Messiahs*, p. 22. Susan Cayleff has pointed out that, despite the fact that women have administered most home remedies across eras and cultures, gender issues have generally been ignored in scholarly interpretations of the patent medicine phenomenon. "Self-Help and the Patent Medicine Business," p. 303.

40. Abbott, "Immigrant and Coal Mining Communities of Illinois," pp. 5–13.

41. Abbott, "Immigrant and Coal Mining Communities," pp. 14–18.

42. Danbom, *Resisted Revolution*, p. 63; McAdam, "The National Menace of Rural Bad Health," p. 321.

43. Philpott, *The Slum and the Ghetto*, pp. 111–21.

44. Hoy, *Chasing Dirt*, p. 119; Chicago Commission on Race Relations, *The Negro in Chicago*, p. 79; Preston and Haines, *Fatal Years*, pp. 209–10.

45. Bonner, *Medicine in Chicago*, pp. 154–56; Beardsley, "Race as a Factor in Health," pp. 124–33. Chicago Community Trust, *Prenatal Care in Chicago*, p. 21. Historian Linda Gordon has made the interesting observation that, in southern states where immigrants constituted less than 2 percent of the population, white women's reform activism was nevertheless also directed at the foreign-born rather than at African Americans. *Pitied But Not Entitled*, p. 111. Other historians have taken the view that intervention by white reformers was not necessarily more advantageous to African Americans than was the virtual neglect of their health care needs. Bruce Bellingham and Mary Pugh Mathis, for example, have argued that white maternal and child health reformers working in the South encouraged African Americans to retain the services of "granny" midwives even though the reformers themselves believed such

services to be medically inferior to those offered by nurses and physicians. See "Race, Citizenship, and the Bio-politics of the Maternalist Welfare State," pp. 157–80.

46. Smith, "'Sick and Tired,'" pp. 18–21; Bonner, *Medicine in Chicago*, pp. 154–56; Hine, *Black Women in White*, pp. 26–31.

47. Smith, "'Sick and Tired,'" pp. 3–5; Hine, "'We Specialize in the Wholly Impossible,'" pp. 70–93.

48. Hine, "'We Specialize in the Wholly Impossible,'" p. 87; Hine, *Black Women in White*, p. 28.

49. Hoy, *Chasing Dirt*, pp. 119–20.

Chapter 2

1. Kingsley, *Steps in the Evolution of Baby Welfare Work*, pp. 6–7.

2. Chicago Visiting Nurse Association, quoted in Burgess, "This Beautiful Charity," p. 60.

3. See, for example, "Infant Mortality and Its Relation to Woman's Employment: A Study of Massachusetts Statistics," Senate Document 645.

4. F. S. Churchill, "Infant Mortality," no page number. Records of the Infant Welfare Society of Chicago, Box 2, folder 2-2.

5. Abbott, *Immigrant and the Community*, p. 145; Kingsley, *Steps in the Evolution of Baby Welfare Work*, p. 6.

6. Helman, *Culture, Health, and Illness*, pp. 45–71. Although the anthropological literature on medicine and culture is vast, relatively few studies have focused on the United States. See, for example, Castro, Furth, and Karlow, "Health Beliefs of Mexican, Mexican American and Anglo American Women"; Eyles and Woods, *Social Geography of Medicine and Health*; Hand, ed., *American Folk Medicine*; Harwood, ed., *Ethnicity and Medical Care*; Pill and Stott, "Concepts of Illness Causation"; Settensen and Colker, "Intercultural Misunderstandings About Health Care"; and Spector, *Cultural Diversity in Health and Illness*.

7. Historian Sandra Schackel has shown that white health reformers working with Hispanic, Indian, and African American mothers in New Mexico enjoyed much more success when they developed a sensitivity to cultural differences among local women and reshaped their own ideas about health and health care to conform to the specific conditions they encountered. Schackel, *Social Housekeepers*, pp. 26–27. Client-centered historical analyses of progressive reform are also found in Gordon, *Heroes of Their Own Lives* and Stadum, *Poor Women and Their Families*.

8. Hamilton, *Exploring the Dangerous Trades*, p. 69; Kingsley, *Steps in the Evolution of Baby Welfare Work*, p. 15; Herzfeld, "Superstitions and Customs of the Tenement-House Mother," p. 985.

9. Hamilton, "Social Settlement and Public Health," p. 1037; Ragucci, "Italian Americans," pp. 230–31.

10. Visiting Nurse Association, *Twenty-third Annual Report* (1912), p. 11.

11. See, for example, Carpenter and Katz, "Study of Acculturation in the Polish

Group of Buffalo"; Jurczak, "Ethnicity, Status, and Generational Positioning"; Kraut, *Silent Travelers*, pp. 105–35; Ragucci, "Generational Continuity and Change," p. 161–62.

12. Interview #WAS-124, Oral History Archives of Chicago Polonia; Porter, "Patient's View," p. 184. To illustrate this point, Antoinette Ragucci cites the Italian proverb "Passata la quarantina, un dolore ogni mattina" (after the age of forty, one can expect a new pain every morning). "Italian Americans," p. 233.

13. Krause, "Urbanization Without Breakdown, " pp. 291–305; McDowell, papers, "An American Citizen in the Making," typescript. Historian James Barrett has shown that Catholic immigrant families in Chicago's Packingtown were willing to go into debt in order to ensure that their children were buried with all the proper observances. Barrett, *Work and Community in the Jungle*, p. 91.

14. Interviews #BAR-080 and #WAS-123, Oral History Archives of Chicago Polonia.

15. *Report of the Health Insurance Commission*, p. 20; Michael Davis, *Immigrant Health and the Community*, pp. 28–29.

16. Witold Kula, Nina Assorodobraj-Kula, and Kula, eds., *Writing Home*, p. 353; Interview #BLA-144, Oral History Archives of Chicago Polonia.

17. Chicago Community Trust, *Eleventh Annual Report of the Elizabeth McCormick Memorial Fund Baby Tents*, June 28–September 11, 1915. Chicago Community Trust, records, Box 27, folder 3.

18. Pehotsky, *Slavic Immigrant Woman*, p. 49; Elizabeth Ewen, *Immigrant Women*, p. 146.

19. Bonner, *Medicine in Chicago*, p. 99; Stevens, *In Sickness and In Wealth*, p. 28; Hedger, "Why the Foreign Woman Does Not Put Her Child in the Hospital," pp. 340–41. Like Dr. Hedger, I have been unable to trace the origin of this particular belief.

20. Interestingly, Kauffman also notes that the drive to modernize and professionalize health care provision that began in the twentieth century resulted in a substantial erosion of this distinctively ethnic dimension within the Catholic hospital environment. Kauffman, *Ministry and Meaning*, pp. 4, 212. A 1903 report found Illinois to have the highest number of Catholic hospitals of any state. Stevens, *In Sickness and In Wealth*, p. 29. Catholic hospitals in relation to philanthropy are discussed by Oates in *Catholic Philanthropic Tradition in America*. On immigrants and Cook County Hospital see Cohen, *Making a New Deal*, p. 63; Bonner, *Medicine in Chicago*, pp. 152–53.

21. Michael Davis, *Immigrant Health and the Community*, pp. 305–42; Rosen, "First Neighborhood Health Center Movement," pp. 475–89.

22. Burgess, "This Beautiful Charity," p. 23.

23. Kingsley, *Steps in the Evolution of Baby Welfare Work*, p. 6.

24. Visiting Nurse Association, *Annual Report* (1913), p. 35; Chicago Community Trust, "1914 Report of the Elizabeth McCormick Memorial Fund Baby Tents,"

Chicago Community Trust, records, Box 27, folder 3.; Visiting Nurse Association, *Annual Report* (1914), p. 13; Visiting Nurse Association, *Annual Report,* (1915), p. 37.

25. Kingsley, *Steps in the Evolution of Baby Welfare Work*, p. 10.

26. Chicago Community Trust, "Baby Welfare Work Summer of 1905." Chicago Community Trust, records, Box 27, folder 3.

27. Chicago Community Trust, "1914 Report of the Elizabeth McCormick Memorial Fund Baby Tents." Chicago Community Trust, records, Box 27, folder 3.

28. Infant Welfare Society of Chicago, Report of the Medical Director for 1911, Henry Booth House, no page number. Infant Welfare Society of Chicago, records, Box 2, folder 2-1.

29. Kauffman, *Ministry and Meaning*, p. 211; Gabaccia, *From the Other Side*, pp. 78–82.

30. Alice Hamilton, "Witchcraft in West Polk Street," pp. 71–75.

31. For an extensive discussion of this worldwide belief, see the essays in Maloney, ed., *Evil Eye*.

32. "Health Customs and Superstitions, " pp. 332–33. Ragucci, "Italian Americans," pp. 226–27.

33. Burgess, "This Beautiful Charity," p. 30; Jurczak, "Ethnicity, Status, and Generational Positioning," pp. 133–34; Ragucci, pp. 238–39; Castro, Furth, and Karlow, "Health Beliefs of Mexican, Mexican American and Anglo American Women," p. 380.

34. Starr, *Social Transformation*, pp. 19–20.

35. DeLee, "Progress Toward Ideal Obstetrics," pp. 114–23; Joint Committee of the Chicago Medical Society and Hull House, "Midwives of Chicago," p. 1346; *Report of the Health Insurance Commission*, p. 60; Interview #KOZ-113, Oral History Archives of Chicago Polonia; Slayton, *Back of the Yards*, p. 73. Historian Nancy Schrom Dye's analysis of records from the New York Midwifery Dispensary shows that working-class women commonly employed a strategy of utilizing both physicians and midwives. "Modern Obstetrics and Working-Class Women," pp. 553–56.

36. Historian Leslie J. Reagan has demonstrated that concern with criminal abortion constituted the major impetus behind progressives' drive to regulate midwifery in Chicago. *When Abortion Was a Crime*, pp. 90–112.

37. Interview #HOJ-066, Oral History Archives of Chicago Polonia. Joint Committee of the Chicago Medical Society and Hull House, "Midwives of Chicago," pp. 1347–49. On the struggle between midwives and other health care practitioners over the control of obstetrical services in the early twentieth century, see Declercq, "Nature and Style of Practice of Immigrant Midwives"; DeVries, *Regulating Birth*; Kobrin, "American Midwife Controversy"; Litoff, *American Midwives*.

38. Burgess, "This Beautiful Charity," p. 30; Michael Davis, *Immigrant Health and the Community*, pp. 131–33.

39. Simkhovitch, *City Worker's World in America*, p. 158; Krasnow, "The Foreigner a Prey of Medical Quacks," pp. 342–46; Michael Davis, *Immigrant Health and*

the Community, pp. 164–67. Historian James Harvey Young argues that the expansion of the market for patent medicines in general owed much to the expansion of the American popular press. *Medical Messiahs*, p. 19. Burgess, "This Beautiful Charity," p. 31.

40. Radzialowski, "'Let Us Join Hands,'" pp. 174–80; Cohen, *Making a New Deal*, p. 62–63; "Medical Lectures for Polish Mothers," *Narod Polski* (July 25, 1917); *L'Italia* (July 13, 1919); "A Word to Mothers," *Dziennik Chicagoski* (May 8–10, 1897) Chicago Foreign Language Press Survey.

41. Michael Davis, *Immigrant Health and the Community*, pp. 145–67.

42. *Saloniki* (May 8, 1905; August 27, 1927) Chicago Foreign Language Press Survey; Michael Davis, *Immigrant Health and the Community*, p. 167.

43. Duffy, *Sanitarians*, p. 208.

44. Visiting Nurse Association, *Thirtieth Annual Report*, p. 15.

45. Visiting Nurse Association, *Twenty-fourth Annual Report*, p. 28; *Twenty-second Annual Report*, p. 40. On the broad mandate of the visiting nurse see Buhler-Wilkerson, *False Dawn* and Reverby, *Ordered to Care*.

46. Burgess, "This Beautiful Charity," p. 131; Visiting Nurse Association, *Twenty-fourth Annual Report*, p. 9.

47. Burgess, "This Beautiful Charity," pp. 146–52; Foley, *Visiting Nurse Manual*, p. 23.

48. Burgess, "This Beautiful Charity," pp. 146–52.

49. Visiting Nurse Association, *Twenty-second Annual Report*, pp. 31, 131; *Twenty-ninth Annual Report*, p. 23.

50. F. S. Churchill, "Studies in Chicago Philanthropy," Infant Welfare Society of Chicago, records, Box 2, folder 2-2; Burgess, "This Beautiful Charity," p. 138; Visiting Nurse Association, "Superintendent's Report," *Twenty-sixth Annual Report*, (1915), p. 30.

51. Infant Welfare Society of Chicago, records. Annual report, 1911.

52. Records of the Infant Welfare Society of Chicago, Box 2, folder 2-2.

53. Reverby, *Ordered to Care*, p. 80.

54. American Child Hygiene Association, "Health Problems of Foreign Born Women and Children," pp. 230–43. In 1919 the American Association for Study and Prevention of Infant Mortality officially changed its name to the American Child Hygiene Association to reflect the expansion of its emphasis on early childhood as well as infancy. See Meckel, *Save the Babies*, p. 202.

55. Hine, *Black Women in White*, p. xv.

56. Burgess, "This Beautiful Charity," pp. 102–4; Visiting Nurse Association, *Thirtieth Annual Report*, p. 14.

57. Alan Kraut has asserted that Italian immigrants from southern provinces brought a long-standing distrust of persons in authority, including doctors and nurses. *Silent Travelers*, p. 135. McDowell, papers, "An American Citizen in the Making," typescript.

58. Hedger, "Report of the Campaign Against Summer Diarrhea," p. 536.

59. Carlson, "Americanization as an Early Twentieth Century Adult Education Movement," pp. 71–72; Barrett, "Americanization from the Bottom Up," pp. 1014–18; McClymer, "Gender and the 'American Way of Life,'" pp. 8–13.

60. American Child Hygiene Association, "Health Problems of Foreign Born Women and Children," pp. 230–43; Van Hoesen, "Relation of the Home-Economics Workers to the Problems of the Foreign Woman," pp. 392–407.

61. Minutes of meetings of Woman's Committee, Council of National Defense, Illinois Division, Book 2. On women in the Americanization movement, see McClymer, "Gender and the 'American Way of Life.'"

62. Hedger, "Problems of the Foreign Mother," p. 56; Sarvasy, "Beyond the Difference versus Equality Debate," p. 355.

63. Brown, "Health Problems of the Foreign Born," p. 103.

64. Michael Davis, *Immigrant Health and the Community*, pp. 8–12. On health reform within the Americanization movement, see also American Child Hygiene Association, *Transactions of the Ninth Annual Meeting*; Department of the Interior, Bureau of Education, *Proceedings, Americanization Conference*; Hbrkova, *Bridging the Atlantic*; Phillip Davis, ed., *Immigration and Americanization*; National Child Welfare Association, "American Citizen."

65. Bessie A. Haasis, "Public Health Nursing, An Agent of Americanization," in *Proceedings of the Americanization Conference*, pp. 381–84.

66. An excellent overview of the Progressive Era drive for legislation to protect women workers is provided by Woloch, introduction to *Muller v. Oregon*, pp. 5–71.

67. Meckel, *Save the Babies*, pp. 186–96; Numbers, *Almost Persuaded*, pp. 75–96.

Chapter 3

1. Streeter, "What? Town Children Healthier Than Ours?" pp. 519–20.

2. Sommers, "Infant Mortality in Rural and Urban Areas," p. 1495–96; Holt, *Linoleum, Better Babies, and the Modern Farm Woman*, pp. 97–98; Preston and Haines, *Fatal Years*, p. 52.

3. Webb, "Good Health," p. 213.

4. Tingley, *Structuring of a State*, pp. 40–43, 284; Hoagland, "The Movement of Rural Population in Illinois," pp. 913–27.

5. *Fourteenth Census*, 365–85; Tingley, *Structuring of a State*, 41.

6. Bevier, Isabel, papers, "Address, January, 1917, Resume of the Report of the Farm Home Survey by Charles L. Stewart"; Bartow, "Rural Water Supplies," pp. 79–84.

7. Tingley, *Structuring of a State*, p. 284; *Fourteenth Census*, pp. 376–85; Shirley J. Carlson, "Black Migration to Pulaski County," pp. 37–46; Jane Adams, *Transformation of Rural Life*, pp. 216–17.

8. "Why Young Women Are Leaving Our Farms," pp. 56–57; Danbom, *Resisted Revolution*, p. 62.

9. Bowers, *The Country Life Movement in America*, pp. 3–5; Jellison, *Entitled to Power*, pp. 1–5; Neth, *Preserving the Family Farm*, pp. 98–106.

10. George Vincent, "Better Health for Rural Communities," p. 19. The Rockefeller Foundation became heavily involved in rural public health issues through its campaign to eradicate hookworm in the South. See Ettling, *Germ of Laziness*.

11. Lathrop, "Address," p. 101.

12. Mitchell, *Dr. George*, p. 346. Rural self-help in medical practice is chronicled in the Rural Illinois Oral History Project, Sangamon State University, Springfield, Illinois. In the 1920s, the Lynds found that the use of home remedies was very much alive in Indiana. *Middletown*, p. 435. See also Hostetler, "Folk Medicine and Sympathy Healing Among the Amish," pp. 249–58. Ella Harvey, "Short Cuts in Family Doctoring," p. 169.

13. "Some Solid Reasons for a Strike of Farm-Wives," pp. 74–78; Clair Adams, *Rural Survey in Illinois*, p. 20.

14. Bane, "Betterment of Living Conditions Among Rural Women," p. 18.

15. Florence Ward, *Farm Woman's Problems*, p. 22. Ward was in charge of extension work with women at the USDA; see Jellison, *Entitled to Power*, pp. 34–37.

16. Jellison, *Entitled to Power*, pp. 5–10.

17. Clair Adams, *Rural Survey in Illinois*, p. 5; "Farm Tenancy in Illinois," pp. 2–3; Jones, *The Dispossessed*, p. 82; George Vincent, "Better Health for Rural Communities," p. 14.

18. Olmsted, "Problems of Maternal Welfare Work in Rural Communities," pp. 207–14.

19. Bevier, papers, "Address, January 1917"; Jellison, *Entitled to Power*, p. 11; Florence Ward, *Farm Woman's Problems*. A discussion of the traditional importance of the rural press within the lives of American country dwellers may be found in Hays, ed., *Early Stories from the Land*, pp. xi–xxii.

20. Health Science Director's Office, Box no. 1, University Archives, University of Illinois at Urbana-Champaign.

21. "Fresh Air," p. 14; Mills, "Proud of Your Baby?" p. 18.

22. "Fly Catechism," p. 13.

23. Rogers, *Dirt and Disease*, p. 7.

24. Carter, "Keep Flies Off Your Baby," p. 19.

25. "Responsibility of Mothers," p. 22.

26. Jellison, *Entitled to Power*, pp. 10–15, 34; "Letters from Our Farm Women," p. 12; Knowles, "'It's Our Turn Now,'" p. 308. An interesting rebuttal to the USDA survey and the responses it publicized is presented in Shepler, "Are Farmers' Wives Neglected and Abused?" p. 3.

27. "What We Ourselves Want," p. 100; Florence Ward, *Farm Woman's Problems*, p. 16.

28. Bailey, "A Study of the Management of the Farm Home," pp. 350–51; Marti, *Women of the Grange*, p. 73.

29. Tilton, "Value of the Country Club," p. 13; A farm woman, "At A Farm

Women's Vacation Camp," p. 7; Warner, "What's the Farm Woman Worth?" p. 12; "Some Solid Reasons for a Strike of Farm-Wives," pp. 74–78.

30. Klaus, *Every Child a Lion*, pp. 238–39. The Children's Bureau's rural studies included Bradley and Williamson, *Rural Children in Selected Counties of North Carolina*; Dart, *Maternity and Child Care in Selected Rural Areas of Mississippi*; Moore, *Maternity and Infant Care in a Rural County in Kansas*; Paradise, *Maternity Care and the Welfare of Young Children in a Homesteading County in Montana*; Sherbon and Moore, *Maternity and Infant Care in Two Rural Counties in Wisconsin*. For an extended discussion and analysis of the letters of rural women to the Children's Bureau, see Molly Ladd-Taylor, *Raising a Baby the Government Way*.

31. Meigs, "Rural Obstetrics," p. 47.

32. Meigs, "Rural Obstetrics," pp. 56–57. A 1919 survey showed that farm wives lived an average of 5.5 miles from the nearest doctor. Knowles, "'It's Our Turn Now,'" p. 313.

33. Meigs, "Rural Obstetrics," p. 56.

34. Anne M. Evans, *Women's Rural Organizations*, pp. 1, 17–18. In 1915, legislation to create a special Farm Women's Bureau in the USDA was introduced into the House of Representatives but never reached the floor of the House. See Knowles, "'It's Our Turn Now,'" pp. 311–12.

35. Neth, *Preserving the Family Farm*, p. 135.

36. Marti, *Women of the Grange*, pp. 5–8, 97; Knowles, "'It's Our Turn Now,'" pp. 312–13.

37. Smith and Wilson, *Agricultural Extension System*, pp. 28–31; Knowles, "'It's Our Turn Now,'" pp. 303–19. Illinois was one of four states to form a women's auxiliary within the Farmers' Institute; nine states organized separate institutes for farm men and farm women. Scott, *Reluctant Farmer*, pp. 120–21.

38. Dunlap, "Address," Champaign County Home Bureau and Home Extension Records; "Mrs. H. Dunlap Started It All," pp. A12–A13.

39. "The State Institute," p. 461; Leonard, "Rural Sanitation," pp. 190–95.

40. Pincomb, papers, 1908–1913, Box 1.; Shapiro, *Perfection Salad*, pp. 188–89; Knowles, "'It's Our Turn Now,'" p. 310.

41. Smith and Wilson, *Agricultural Extension System*, pp. 59–69, 192–93; Bane, *The County Home Bureau in Illinois*, p. 4; Wilson, Smith, and Burns, *Measuring the Progress of Extension Work*, p. 3.

42. "Let Us Counsel Together," p. 78; Jellison, *Entitled to Power*, p. 21; Bane, *Story of Isabel Bevier*, p. 60. Counties with Home Bureaus in 1919 were Adams, Champaign, Hancock, Kane, Kankakee, LaSalle, Livingston, Logan, McHenry, McLean, Macon, Madison, Mercer, Saline, Tazewell, Vermilion, and Williamson. "Home and Household," p. 30; Bane, papers, "Home Economics Extension Service in Illinois," typescript, n.d., Box 1.

43. Shapiro, *Perfection Salad*, p. 218; Knowles, "'It's Our Turn Now,'" pp. 314–15. Bunch, "A Course for Home Demonstration Agents," p. 431. Bunch was State Leader of Home Extension Services for Illinois.

44. Fink, *Agrarian Women*, pp. 131–35; Jellison, *Entitled to Power*, pp. 21–23, 62; Esposito, *Places of Pride*, pp. 12–15; McKinney, "Clara Brian," p. 4.

45. Letter dated November 20, 1909 from J. B. Burrows to Eugene Davenport, Dean of the College of Agriculture, University of Illinois. Bevier, papers, Box 1.; Bane, *Story of Isabel Bevier*, pp. 58–59; Shapiro, *Perfection Salad*, pp. 184–85; Knowles, "'It's Our Turn Now,'" p. 311.

46. Jellison, *Entitled to Power*, 37; Neth, *Preserving the Family Farm*, pp. 135–38; Jensen, introduction, to *Promise to the Land*, pp. 1–28.

47. Bane, papers, "Bane, Lita — Personal History" and "Notes for Talks Regarding Home Economics," n.d., Box 1; Bevier, papers, "Outlook and Adjustment Conferences Material, 1928–1929," Box 2; Esposito, *Places of Pride*, pp. 15–17. The USDA reported that the cost of installing a plumbing system in the "typical" Iowa farm house was $300. Jellison, *Entitled to Power*, p. 39.

48. See, for example, Cowan, *More Work for Mother*; Hayden, *Grand Domestic Revolution*; Strasser, *Never Done*.

49. The fifteen northern Home Bureau counties were: Adams, Champaign, Hancock, Kane, Kankakee, LaSalle, Livingston, Logan, McHenry, McLean, Macon, Madison, Mercer, Tazewell, and Vermilion. The southern Home Bureau counties were Saline and Williamson. "Home and Household," p. 30. Wilson, Smith, and Burns, *Measuring the Progress of Home Extension Work*, pp. 12–13.

50. *The Extension News* 1 (April, 1919). Agricultural Extension News and Extension Notes, Box 1; *The Home Bureau Bulletin* 6 (August and November 1926). Champaign County Home Bureau Records.

51. Bane, *Story of Isabel Bevier*, 59; *Home Bureau Bulletin* I (December 1919), Champaign County Home Bureau Records; "First Schools," p. 1.

Chapter 4

1. "An Effective Exhibition of a Community Survey," p. 100.

2. Russell Sage Foundation, *The Springfield Survey*, pp. 371–76.

3. On changes in midwestern rural culture see Kirschner, *City and Country*, pp. 252–57. Historian John Ettling has described the health reform activities sponsored by the Rockefeller Sanitary Commission in its antihookworm campaign in the rural South as drawing from — and exploiting — the region's tent revival tradition. *Germ of Laziness*, pp. 162–63.

4. Miller and Montgomery, *A Chautauqua to Remember*, p. 105.

5. See *Infant Feeding*; "Publications of the State Board of Health," p. 37. It is interesting to note that the Illinois public health pamphlet on infant care actually predates the better-known publication distributed by the U.S. Children's Bureau. *Infant Care* was first published in 1914, two years after the bureau's founding. On Children's Bureau publications and their role in national child health campaigns see Ladd-Taylor, *Raising a Baby the Government Way*.

6. "Board of Health Reissues Circular," pp. 100–101; "The Care of Babies," p. 98; "Our Babies," p. 11; East, *Better Baby Conference*, p. 22.

7. Ruediger, "Program of Public Health, " pp. 235–47; Eldridge, *Social Legislation in Illinois*, pp. 57–58.

8. "Flora To Have Better Baby Week." I am grateful to Calvin Clay Snyder for bringing the latter news item to my attention; "Baby Week in Illinois," p. 105; Klaus, *Every Child a Lion*, pp. 137–38, 234.

9. Jellison, *Entitled to Power*, p. 54. Extension activities created a huge bureaucracy in the USDA; in the period from 1890 to 1920, the department's size increased by more than thirtyfold. Fink, *Agrarian Women*, p. 27.

10. Bevier, papers, Box 1, "Household Science Extension Report, 1915–1916" and "1916–1917" and "Home Economics Extension Report, 1916–1917."

11. Bevier, papers, "Home Economics Extension Report, 1917–1918," Box 1, and "Outlook and Adjustment Conferences Material, 1928–1929," Box 2.

12. Champaign County Home Bureau and Home Extension Records, *Home Bureau Bulletin* 6 (August 1926) and *Home Bureau Bulletin* 6 (November 1926); *Extension News* 1 (November 1918) and *Agricultural Extension News* 12 (November 1930).

13. "Foreword," *Illinois Health News* 1 (January 1915), p. 1.

14. Rawlings, *Rise and Fall of Disease in Illinois*, pp. 134–35, 174–94, 234–35; Bonner, *Medicine in Chicago*, p. 191; Rosen, *Preventive Medicine*, pp. 22–23; "New State Department of Public Health," pp. 83–84.

15. Bonner, *Medicine in Chicago*, p. 191; "Exhibit Material for Baby Week," pp. 69–71.

16. "State Board of Health Exhibit," pp. 35–43.

17. East, *Better Baby Conference*, pp. 20–22.

18. Ewen and Ewen, *Channels of Desire*, pp. 82–87; Gomery, *Shared Pleasures*, pp. 29–30; Neth, *Preserving the Family Farm*, p. 255.

19. Hammer, *Recreation in Springfield*, pp. 39–41, 80–82; *Woman's City Club Bulletin* (May 1917): 9.

20. May, *Screening Out the Past*, p. 52; Sloan, *Loud Silents*, pp. 4–11; "Worthy Exhibit," p. 2; "Without Proof," *Illinois Health News* 2, back cover; "Better Babies," pp. 69–70; Rawlings, *Rise and Fall of Disease in Illinois*, pp. 177–78; East, *Better Baby Conference*, p. 21. An extensive repository of early public health films is housed at the Historical Health Film Collection at the University of Michigan, Ann Arbor. I am grateful to Martin Pernick for sharing information about the collection with me.

21. Klaus, *Every Child a Lion*, pp. 144–57; Holt, *Linoleum, Better Babies, and the Modern Farm Woman*, pp. 112–14; "Better Babies," p. 55.

22. Downey, "Have You a 'Better Baby'?" p. 7.

23. "Better Babies," pp. 53–55; Illinois State Department of Agriculture, "Better Baby Contests," *State Fair Annual Report*, 1919, pp. 356–58. On the development of normative physical standards for children, see Woodbury, *Statures and Weights of Children Under Six Years of Age*. Historian Joan Jacobs Brumberg has noted the increasing tendency in this period to associate lower-than-average weight in children

with lower-class status. *Fasting Girls*, p. 237. Klaus describes the "psychological tests" given to better baby conference participants in Oregon. *Every Child a Lion*, p. 148.

24. "Better Babies," pp. 55, 65–69; East, *Better Baby Conference*, pp. 14–19; "Fifth Annual Better Babies Conference," pp. 69–74; Illinois Farmers' Institute, *Yearbook 1916*, p. 69.

25. "Better Babies," p. 57.

26. Illinois State Department of Agriculture, *State Fair Annual Report*, 1919, p. 360.

27. Mills, "Proud of Your Baby?" p. 18; Gear, "Baby's Picture," pp. 419–42.

28. "Fifth Annual Better Babies Conference," p. 70.

29. "Better Babies," p. 53; "Demonstrations and Better Baby Conferences," p. 291; Klaus, *Every Child a Lion*, pp. 156–57.

30. "Fifth Annual Better Babies Conference," pp. 71–74; Klaus, *Every Child a Lion*, pp. 149–51.

31. Holt, *Linoleum, Better Babies, and the Modern Farm Woman*, p. 115; Blee, *Women of the Klan*, pp. 20, 187 n. 25.

32. Pernick, *Black Stork*, pp. 48–54. Holt, *Linoleum, Better Babies, and the Modern Farm Woman*, p. 113; Illinois State Department of Agriculture, *State Fair Annual Report*, 1921, p. 31c.

33. Downey, "Have You a 'Better Baby'?" p. 7.

34. Meigs, "Infant Welfare Work in Wartime," p. 83.

35. "Caroline Hedger," *Who's Who in Chicago*, p. 399; "Welcome to Women in Public Health Work," p. 164; McDowell, "Mothers and Night Work," p. 335.

36. Collections of the Infant Welfare Society of Chicago, Box 1, folder 1-1; "Chicago's Baby Week," p. 296 In April 1914, President Woodrow Wilson, upon learning that a German munitions ship was due to land at Veracruz, ordered the occupation of that Mexican port city to prevent weapons from reaching the government of Victoriano Huerta, who had seized power and murdered President Francisco Madero a few months earlier. A skirmish ensued in which 400 Mexican soldiers were killed. See Link, *Wilson*, pp. 232–66.

37. Jenison, "The War-Time Organization of Illinois," pp. 39–41; Bowen, "War Work of the Women of Illinois," pp. 322–23; Minutes of meetings of Woman's Committee, Book I; Estelle Frances Ward, "Practical Patriotism," p. 556. Louise de Koven Bowen served as the most important single financial benefactor of Hull House. Sklar, "Who Funded Hull House?" pp. 94–115; "Bowen, Louise de Koven (Mrs. Joseph Tilton B.)," Marquis, ed., *Book of Chicagoans*, p. 77.

38. Jenison, *War Documents and Addresses*, p. 127; Estelle Frances Ward, "Practical Patriotism," pp. 557–58; Bowen, "War Work of the Women of Illinois," pp. 322–23; Lemons, *Woman Citizen*, p. 5; Muncy, *Creating a Female Dominion*, p. 99.

39. *Seventh Annual Report of the Chief, Children's Bureau*; *Final Report of the Woman's Committee*, p. 156.

40. "Welcome to Women in Public Health Work," p. 164; Records of the Infant

Welfare Society of Chicago, Box 1, folder 1; Cudahy, "Report of Nurses Committee for 1918," pp. 12–15; Estelle Frances Ward, "Practical Patriotism," pp. 556–57; "Wood, Alice Holabird (Mrs. Ira Couch Wood)," Marquis, ed., *Book of Chicagoans*, p. 741.

41. Records of the Infant Welfare Society of Chicago, Box 8, folder 8-1. The complete list of affiliated organizations is as follows: Illinois State Department of Public Health, Illinois State Department of Public Welfare, Society for the Prevention of Tuberculosis, States' Relations Service of the Department of Agriculture, University of Illinois, Federation of Women's Clubs, State Parent-Teachers Association, Federation of Labor, Cook County League of Clubs, Catholic Woman's League, Pediatric Society, Federation of Day Nurseries, Infant Welfare Society of Chicago, Juvenile Protective Association, Chicago Board of Education, Vocational Guidance Bureau, Visiting Nurse Association, Chicago Woman's Aid, Jewish Aid Society, Illinois Children's Home and Aid Society, Red Cross Teaching Center, Woman's City Club, Chicago Medical Association, Illinois Medical Association, Chicago Political Equity League, Central Council of Social Agencies, Cook County Bureau of Social Service, Cook County Country Life Directors, Illinois Society for the Prevention of Blindness. *Final Report of the Woman's Committee*, p. 154.

42. Ibid., pp. 150–59.

43. Ibid., pp. 171–75.

44. Ibid., pp. 180–83.

45. "Illinois State Fair Notes," p. 1674; Rawlings, *Rise and Fall of Disease in Illinois*, p. 237; Illinois State Department of Agriculture, *Illinois State Fair Annual Report, 1921*, pp. 309–10.

46. "Better Babies Contest Most Successful Ever Held," p. 223.

47. "Seventh Annual Better Babies Conference," p. 291; "Reviving County Fair," p. 34; "Better Babies Conferences Conducted in 1922," p. 97.

48. Paulson, papers, "County Problems Outside of Decatur," folder 8, "ARC Central Division, Macon Co. IL Survey Reports," typescript, n.d. The American Red Cross rural surveys under Paulson's supervision were conducted between 1919 and 1920. Waller, *Main Street Amusements*, pp. 238–39.

49. American Association for Study and Prevention of Infant Mortality, *Transactions of the Ninth Annual Meeting*, p. 232. Some historians have emphasized the beneficial effects of wartime enthusiasm for progressive reforms in the United States and England. See, for example, Davis, *Spearheads for Reform*; Wynn, *From Progressivism to Prosperity*; Dwork, *War Is Good for Babies*.

50. See, for example, Kennedy, *Over Here*; Hawley, *Great War and the Search for a Modern Order*; Link and McCormick, eds., *Progressivism*; Rodgers, "In Search of Progressivism"; Wiebe, *Search for Order*.

Chapter 5

1. *Chicago Daily News*, March 19, 1923. The Sheppard-Towner Act has attracted the attention of scholars interested in the historical development of the Amer-

ican welfare state. See, for example, Chepaitis, "First Federal Social Welfare Measure"; Costin, *Two Sisters for Social Justice*; Gordon, *Pitied But Not Entitled*; Klaus, *Every Child a Lion*; Koven and Michel, eds., *Mothers of a New World*; Ladd-Taylor, *Mother-Work*; Lemons, *Woman Citizen*; Muncy, *Creating a Female Dominion*; Reilinger, "Child Health and the State." Theda Skocpol has argued that the Sheppard-Towner Act put into effect the maternalist vision of national well-being through preventive health care. *Protecting Soldiers and Mothers*, p. 512.

2. "Committee on Child Welfare," p. 18; "Infant Welfare in Moline," p. 124.

3. Illinois League of Women Voters, *First Ten Years*, p. 6.

4. Meckel, *Save the Babies*, p. 210; Sklar, "Historical Foundations of Women's Power," pp. 43–93; Ladd-Taylor, *Mother-Work*, pp. 167–96; Lemons, *Woman Citizen*, pp. 153–80; Muncy, *Creating a Female Dominion*, pp. 93–132; Skocpol, *Protecting Soldiers and Mothers*, pp. 480–524.

5. Buechler, *Transformation of the Women's Suffrage Movement*; Wheeler, *Roads They Made*, pp. 107–8.

6. Meckel identifies each of these factors as deleterious to Sheppard-Towner on the national level as well. *Save the Babies*, p. 207.

7. *Report of the Health Insurance Commission of the State of Illinois*, p. 46. The commission's members, appointed by Governor Lowden, included representatives of labor, employers, farmers, physicians, and attorneys as well as Chicago health reform activists Alice Hamilton and Edna Foley. Bennett, "The Movement for Compulsory Health Insurance," p. 237.

8. The national agencies that participated in the Springfield survey were: American Association of Societies for Organizing Charity, National Association for the Study and Prevention of Tuberculosis, National Committee for Mental Hygiene, National Housing Association, and the United States Public Health Service. State organizations were: Illinois Conference of Charities and Corrections, Illinois State Board of Health, Illinois State Department of Factory Inspection, Illinois State Food Commission, and the Illinois State Water Survey. "An Effective Exhibition of a Community Survey," pp. 95–100.

9. Russell Sage Foundation, *Springfield Survey*, pp. 25, 138.

10. Ibid., pp. 216–22, 238–40, 243, 251–53.

11. Rawlings, *Rise and Fall*, pp. 182, 234–35; "Examination and Licensure of Physicians," p. 197; Pegram, *Partisans and Progressives*, pp. 198–200; "New State Department of Public Health," p. 84. Under the 1917 reorganization, the Illinois State Board of Health officially became the Illinois State Department of Public Health.

12. "Dr. Rawlings Appointed Director," p. 1.

13. "Important Health Legislation Fails," p. 1; Rawlings, "Adequate Provision for Public Health," p. 143; Rawlings, *Rise and Fall*, pp. 194–95; Nauss, "Health Activities in Rural Illinois," pp. 121–31.

14. Transcript of interview with Dr. Isaac D. Rawlings, dated March 7, [1924?]. Illinois League of Women Voters, records, Box 3, folder 14.

15. Children's Bureau, *Promotion of the Welfare and Hygiene of Maternity and Infancy*, CB publication no. 137, Washington: Government Printing Office, 1924.

16. Letter from Isaac Rawlings to Grace Abbott, June 7, 1922. Illinois League of Women Voters, collections, Box 7, folder 52.

17. For contemporary descriptions of the work of rural public health nurses in the Midwest, see Brainard, *Evolution of Public Health Nursing*, passim, and Fox, "Rural Public Health Nursing," pp. 67–77. Historian Darlene Clark Hine has asserted that African American public health nurses often represented the sole source of medical care for many black communities in the rural South. Hine, *Black Women in White*, pp. 154–55.

18. "Illinois Agreement of Public Health Nursing," pp. 163–65; "Directory of Public Health Nurses of Illinois," pp. 228–31.

19. Rawlings to Abbott, June 7, 1922. Illinois League of Women Voters, collections, Box 7, folder 52.

20. Rawlings to Abbott, June 7, 1922. Illinois League of Women Voters, collections, Box 7, folder 52.

21. Children's Bureau, *Promotion of Welfare and Hygiene*, pp. 3–4.

22. Bonner, *Medicine in Chicago*, p. 189; "Evans, William A.," *Who's Who in Chicago*, p. 281. Although Illinois finally qualified as a U.S. birth registration area beginning in 1923, as of June 1922, 59 counties still had not met the federal requirements for 90 percent accuracy in birth registration. "How the Counties Stood in Federal Birth Registration Test," no page number.

23. Minutes of the Conference on the Sheppard-Towner Act, June 21, 1922. Illinois League of Women Voters, collections, Box 7, folder 52. Thomas R. Pegram has described the distrust that small farmers in Illinois displayed toward both an expanding government structure and the large farm operators in the state. Pegram, "Public Health and Progressive Dairying in Illinois," pp. 36–51.

24. "Statistics averaged for 1920 and 1921." Illinois League of Women Voters, collections, Box 7, folder 52.

25. Letter from Isaac Rawlings to Edith Rockwood, December 5, 1922. Illinois League of Women Voters, Box 7, folder 52.

26. "Statistics averaged for 1920 and 1921." Illinois League of Women Voters, Box 7, folder 52.

27. "Sheppard-Towner Conference, November 20, 1922," typescript. Illinois League of Women Voters, Box 7, folder 53.

28. "Objections to the Sheppard-Towner Bill," p. 143.

29. See "Reject Humiliating Federal Aid."

30. "Sheppard-Towner Bill as Amended is as Bad as the Original Bill," pp. 471–72; Bonner, *Medicine in Chicago*, pp. 205, 219.

31. "An Act for the Promotion of the Welfare and Hygiene of Maternity and Infancy," Section 8. The full text of the act is cited in Chepaitis, "First Federal Social Welfare Measure," pp. 370–74; conservative opposition to Sheppard-Towner and the

resultant amendment to the original bill is described in Meckel, *Save the Babies*, pp. 200–15.

32. Numbers, *Almost Persuaded*, pp. 106–7. A different perspective on the changing relationship between physicians and the state is offered by Reagan, "About to Meet Her Maker," pp. 1240–1264.

33. In *Massachusetts v. Mellon*, plaintiffs charged that the legislation both violated the rights of individual taxpayers and threatened to destroy local self-government by extending the power of the federal government into maternity and infant care, a purely local matter. The court dismissed the suit, but Justice Sutherland's comments made it clear that the Sheppard-Towner Act presented no constitutional problems because individual states could retain all of their prerogatives simply by refusing to participate in the program. The Court's position in *Massachusetts v. Mellon* set an important precedent for subsequent federal programs using the grants-in-aid structure. Urofsky, ed., "Massachusetts v. Mellon," pp. 132–34; Chepaitis, "First Federal Social Welfare Measure," pp. 182–209; Skocpol, *Protecting Soldiers and Mothers*, pp. 506–7.

34. While the flexing of their political muscles represented a relatively new stance for both the AMA and the ISMS, historian Thomas Neville Bonner has demonstrated that, as early as the 1890s, the organized medical profession perceived its own interests to be in harmony with those of the commercial and industrial leaders in the state. Bonner, *Medicine in Chicago*, pp. 205, 219. See also Numbers, *Almost Persuaded*, pp. 75–96, 107; Lemons, *Woman Citizen*, p. 163; Chepaitis, "First Federal Social Welfare Measure," p. 103.

35. Numbers, *Almost Persuaded*, pp. 9–10; Rothman, "Women's Clinics or Doctors' Offices," pp. 175–201; Burrow, *Organized Medicine in the Progressive Era*, pp. 111–12; Daniel Fox, *Health Policies, Health Politics*, p. 15; Meckel, *Save the Babies*, p. 217; Rosenkrantz, *Public Health and the State*, pp. 131–33.

36. Numbers, *Almost Persuaded*, p. 97; Bennett, "Movement for Compulsory Health Insurance in Illinois," pp. 233–46; "Governor Lowden Approves of State Medical Society Resolution," p. 424; Bonner, *Medicine in Chicago*, p. 246.

37. Whalen, "Abuse of Medical Charities in Chicago," pp. 1–7; "Health Centers Not Needed in Illinois," pp. 262–64; Chicago Community Trust, *Prenatal Care in Chicago*, pp. 95–96.

38. Foley, *Visiting Nurse Manual*, pp. 33–34.

39. "Is the Nurse Jeopardizing the Public Health Service?" pp. 129–30.

40. "Objections to the Sheppard-Towner Maternity Bill," p. 132.

41. Illinois General Assembly, "House Bill 298," *House Bills* 2, 1923–1924, and "Senate Bill 175," *Senate Bills* 1, 1912.

42. Pegram, *Partisans and Progressives*, p. 10.

43. "Interview with Speaker Shanahan 1/22/23," typescript, Illinois League of Women Voters, Box 7, folder 52; telephone message from Grace Meigs Crowder to the ILWV. ILWV, Box 7, folder 52.

44. Collections of the Illinois League of Women Voters, Box 7, folder 52.

45. See "Decision Upholds Maternity Act." For discussions of the Chicago Archdiocese's initiatives in social reform under the leadership of Cardinal Mundelein, see Dolan, *American Catholic Experience*; Kennelly, *American Catholic Women*; Shanabruch, *Chicago's Catholics.*

46. "National Maternity Bill," *Farmer's Wife* 33 (November 1921): 529. *The Farmer's Wife* also published a very supportive editorial on Julia Lathrop's work as chief of the Children's Bureau upon her retirement, *Farmer's Wife* 33 (November 1921): 595. Historian Alisa Klaus has observed that Children's Bureau officials tended to demonstrate more gender solidarity and sympathy when working with white rural women than they did with either urban immigrants or African American women. Klaus, *Every Child a Lion*, pp. 230–31. Ladd-Taylor has argued that the Children's Bureau, in fact, had the nation's rural areas specifically in mind when it designed the Sheppard-Towner plan. Ladd-Taylor, *Mother-Work*, pp. 187–88; Jellison, *Entitled to Power*, pp. 7–8. More recently, historians Bruce Bellingham and Mary Pugh Mathis have argued that Sheppard-Towner programs in the rural South actually perpetuated institutionalized racism by setting up medicalized maternity care for white women while consigning African American women to the care of lay midwives. "Race, Citizenship and Bio-politics of the Maternalist Welfare State," pp. 157–80.

47. United States Children's Bureau, *Directory of Local Child-Health Agencies*, pp. 89–93.

48. *Illinois Farmers' Institute, Department of Household Science, Yearbook 1923*, p. 186.

49. Letter from J. B. DeLee to Alice Wood, May 5, 1923. Illinois League of Women Voters, Box 7, folder 53.

50. "Another Word on the Maternity Bill," typescript, n.d. Illinois League of Women Voters, collections, Box 7, folder 54. In addition to Hedger and Evans, the group included Charles M. Bacon (general practice), William Francis Hewitt (obstetrics and gynecology), Henry William Cheney (pediatrician), and Clifford Grulee (pediatrician). Hewitt taught medicine at Rush Medical College; Cheney and Grulee taught at Northwestern University. Another signer, James A. Britton, was the husband of Gertrude Howe Britton, a Hull House resident and director of social services at the Central Free Dispensary of Rush Medical College. Albert Nelson Marquis, ed., *Who's Who in Chicago* (Chicago: A. N. Marquis, 1926). The other physicians who signed the document were Theresa K. Jennings, Josephine Milligan, Harold A. Rosenbaum, Eva M. Wilson, and Frank Walls Young.

51. Letter from Alice Wood, April 2, 1923. Illinois League of Women Voters, collections, Box 7, folder 53.

52. "Federal Aid to States a Real Menace," p. 357; "Delusion of Federal Aid." Lathrop is quoted in Muncy, *Creating a Female Dominion*, p. 132.

53. Numbers, *Almost Persuaded*, p. 77; "In Memoriam," pp. 358–59; "Government Operation Always Costly," p. 59.

54. "Maternity Legislation is Paternalistic and Socialistic," p. 375; "Who is Responsible for the Sheppard-Towner Maternity Bill?" pp. 414–15. Historians Sonya Michel and Robyn Rosen point out the irony that women working in these virulently antigovernment organizations became extremely skillful at exploiting both state and national legislatures. "The Paradox of Maternalism," p. 375.

55. Bonner, *Medicine in Chicago*, p. 222.

56. "Russian Maternity System," p. 6. A "spider's web" chart, purporting to show the links between prominent women reformers including Jane Addams, Julia Lathrop, and Grace Abbott with Bolshevist leaders in Moscow, was originally printed in the *Woman Patriot* and reprinted by the ultraconservative press. Many of the editorials featuring the chart implicated American women reformers in an international conspiracy to take over the United States. Lemons, *Woman Citizen*, pp. 209–27; Costin, *Two Sisters for Social Justice*, pp. 143–46.

57. Ladd-Taylor, *Mother-Work*, pp. 167–69. For a more general discussion on the post-World War I conservative backlash against Chicago settlement house reformers see Carson, *Settlement Folk*; Fitzpatrick, *Endless Crusade*; Graham, *Great Campaigns*; McClymer, *War and Welfare*.

58. Reprinted in Bremner, *Children and Youth in America*, pp. 1019–20; "Soviet Feature of the Sheppard Maternity Bill," pp. 263–64.

59. "Objections to the Sheppard-Towner Maternity Bill," p. 132. On professional conflicts between physicians and nurses in this era see Melosh, *Physician's Hand*, passim.

60. "Why Illinois Should Not Cooperate," p. 176; "Should the Whole Family Be Eligible Under Mothers' Pension Laws?" p. 265.

61. Letter from Mabel M. Dunlap to Mrs. Kenneth Rich, February 19, 1923. Illinois League of Women Voters, Box 7, folder 52.

62. Chepaitis, "First Federal Social Welfare Measure," p. 162.

63. Fifty-third General Assembly, State of Illinois. *Senate Debates*, pp. 577–90; "Senate Vote on the Sheppard-Towner Cooperation Bill," pp. 409–10. *Legislative Synopsis and Digest* (1923), pp. 55–56, 239; *Journal of the Senate* (1923), pp. 448, 712–15, 784, 908–9; "Assembly Will Adjourn Today," p. 1.

64. Typescript of notes on interviews with physicians, March–April 1924. Collections of the Illinois League of Women Voters, Box 3, folder 14. Rawlings omitted all but the most oblique of references to Sheppard-Towner in his volume commemorating the fiftieth anniversary of the State Department of Public Health. Rawlings, *Rise and Fall*, passim.

65. Leigh, *Federal Health Administration*, p. 423; "Editorial," *Survey* 58 (April 15, 1927): 80.

66. Numbers, *Almost Persuaded*, p. 27; Chepaitis, "First Federal Social Welfare Measure," pp. 215–77; Costin, *Two Sisters for Social Justice*, pp. 147–48; Ladd-Taylor, *Mother-Work*, pp. 184–90; Lemons, *Woman Citizen*, pp. 209–27; Meckel, *Save the Babies*, pp. 200–219; Muncy, *Creating a Female Dominion*, pp. 126–57.

67. Pegram, *Partisans and Progressives*, pp. xii, 23; Flanagan, "Exercising New Rights."

68. Pegram, *Partisans and Progressives*, pp. xii, 205; Tingley, *Structuring of a State*, pp. 372–74; Bonner, *Medicine in Chicago*, p. 194.

69. Rawlings, *Rise and Fall*, p. 199; "Summary of Child Hygiene Activities," p. 175.

70. Keating, "Infant Welfare Society Practicing Medicine," pp. 279–81. See also Daniel Fox, *Health Policies, Health Politics*, p. 15; Meckel, *Save the Babies*, p. 217; Stevens, *American Medicine and the Public Interest*, pp. 142–45.

71. Stevens, *In Sickness and In Wealth*, pp. 106–22; Rosen, "First Neighborhood Health Center Movement," pp. 475–89; Rosenberg, "Social Class and Medical Care," pp. 273–85; Buhler-Wilkerson, *False Dawn*, pp. 195–219; Hine, *Black Women in White*, p. 31; Bonner, *Medicine in Chicago*, p. 139.

72. Streeter, "Where's the Doctor When You Need Him?" p. 15; Kirkpatrick, *Farmer's Standard of Living*, p. 179.

73. United States Bureau of the Census: *Thirteenth Census* 4; *Fourteenth Census* 6; *Fifteenth Census* 4. Published census tables for the years 1910, 1920, and 1930 enumerated the number of physicians in towns of between 25,000 and 100,000 residents, but not for those living in rural areas (defined as less than 2,500 residents).

74. Steadman, *Public Health Organization*, p. 149.

75. United States Bureau of the Census, *Sixteenth Census* 3; Mott and Roemer, *Rural Health and Medical Care*, p. 158. Historian Michael R. Grey argues that the Farm Security Administration's decision to organize medical cooperatives in 1935 resulted from the fact that expenses for illness and injury represented a major reason why farmers defaulted on their loans. Grey, "Poverty, Politics, and Health," pp. 320–50.

76. Rawlings, *Rise and Fall*, p. 200.

Epilogue

1. Lentzner, "Seasonal Patterns," pp. 8–9; Preston and Haines, *Fatal Years*, pp. 208–10; Meckel, "Judging Progressive Era Infant Welfare," pp. 105–12; Antler and Fox, "Movement toward a Safe Maternity," pp. 490–506.

2. Illinois State Planning Commission, *Infant Mortality in Illinois*, p. 1. Figures for the years 1900 to 1906 are not available for the state of Illinois as a whole due to the inconsistent record-keeping practices of that period; Illinois in fact, did not qualify for the U.S. birth registration area until 1923.

3. United States Bureau of the Census, *Fourteenth Census* 4, pp. 365–85; Tingley, *Structuring of a State*, p. 41. Anthropologist Jane Adams had observed that substantial class and status variations existed among residents of Union County in southern Illinois during the 1920s and 1930s. Adams, *Transformation of Rural Life*, pp. 132–43.

4. "Northern Babies Fare Best," pp. 253–59.

5. Vinikas, *Soft Soap, Hard Sell*, pp. 82–83. Historian T. J. Jackson Lears argues that advertisers were well aware of women's central responsibility for maintaining both their family's health and its social respectability, and advertising trade journals emphasized the importance of reaching a female audience when promoting new personal and domestic hygiene products. Lears, "From Salvation to Self-Realization," pp. 5–38; Apple, *Vitamania*, pp. 18–25; Stewert Ewen, *Captains of Consciousness*, pp. 169–70; Harvey Green, *Uncertainty of Everyday Life*, pp. 184–185. Hayden, *Grand Domestic Revolution*, pp. 284–86.

BIBLIOGRAPHY

Manuscript Collections

Agricultural Extension News and Extension Notes. University of Illinois at Urbana-Champaign Archives, Urbana, Illinois.

Bane, Juliet Lita, papers. University of Illinois at Urbana-Champaign Archives, Urbana, Illinois.

Bevier, Isabel, papers. University of Illinois at Urbana-Champaign Archives, Urbana, Illinois.

Champaign County Home Bureau and Home Extension Records. Champaign County Historical Society Archives, Urbana, Illinois.

Chicago Community Trust, records. Chicago Historical Society, Chicago, Illinois.

Chicago Foreign Language Press Survey. Microfilm, University of Illinois at Urbana-Champaign Library, Urbana, Illinois.

Douglas County Home Bureau, records. Douglas County Historical Association, Tuscola, Illinois.

Elizabeth McCormick Memorial Fund, records. Midwest Women's History Collection, University of Illinois, Chicago.

Health Science Director's Office. University of Illinois at Urbana-Champaign Archives, Urbana, Illinois.

Illinois League of Women Voters, records. Chicago Historical Society, Chicago, Illinois.

Illinois State Department of Agriculture, State Fair Annual Reports. Record Group 201.003, Illinois State Archives, Springfield, Illinois.

Infant Welfare Society of Chicago, records. Chicago Historical Society, Chicago, Illinois.

McDowell, Mary, papers. Chicago Historical Society, Chicago, Illinois.

Oral History Archives of Chicago Polonia. Chicago Historical Society, Chicago, Illinois.

Paulson, Evalina Beldin, papers. Midwest Women's History Collection, University of Illinois at Chicago.

Pincomb, Helena M., papers, 1908–1913. University of Illinois at Urbana-Champaign Archives, Urbana, Illinois.

Rural Illinois Oral History Project. University of Illinois at Springfield.

United States Marine Hospital Service (Cairo, Illinois), records, 1877–1936. Illinois State Historical Library, Springfield, Illinois.

Visiting Nurse Association of Chicago, records. Chicago Historical Society, Chicago, Illinois.

Woman's Committee, Council of National Defense, Illinois Division, records. Illinois State Archives, Springfield, Illinois.

Primary Sources

Abbott, Grace. "The Immigrant and Coal Mining Communities of Illinois." *Bulletin of the Immigrants Commission* 2 (1920): 5–13.

———. *The Immigrant and the Community.* New York: Century, 1917.

Adams, Clair S. *A Rural Survey of Illinois.* New York: Board of Home Missions of the Presbyterian Church in the U.S.A., n.d.

American Association for Study and Prevention of Infant Mortality. *Transactions of the Ninth Annual Meeting* (1918). Baltimore: Franklin Printing, 1919.

American Child Hygiene Association. *Transactions of the Ninth Annual Meeting, Chicago, December 5–7, 1919.* Baltimore: Franklin Printing, 1919.

Annual Report of the Illinois State Board of Health, 1902–1913. Springfield: Illinois State Board of Health, 1914.

"Assembly Will Adjourn Today. Many Bills Die." *Illinois State Journal* (June 19, 1923). Springfield, Illinois.

"Baby Week in Illinois." *Illinois Health News* 2 (1916): 105–6.

Bailey, Ilena. "A Study of the Management of the Farm Home." *Journal of Home Economics* 7 (August–September 1915): 348–53.

Bane, Juliet Lita. "Betterment of Living Conditions Among Rural Women." M.A. thesis, University of Chicago, 1919.

———. *The County Home Bureau in Illinois.* Urbana: University of Illinois Agricultural College and Experiment Station, 1922.

Bartow, Edward. "Rural Water Supplies." *Chemical and Biological Survey of the Waters of Illinois.* University of Illinois Bulletin, Water Survey Series no. 7 (September 1909).

"Better Babies: Suggestions for Organizing and Conducting Baby Health Conferences." *Illinois Health News* 3 (1917): 53–55.

"Better Babies Conferences Conducted in 1922." *Illinois Health News* 9 (1923): 97.

"Better Babies Contest Most Successful Ever Held." *Illinois Health News* 7 (1921): 223.

"Board of Health Reissues Circular." *Illinois State Board of Health Bulletin* 5 (1909): 100–101.

The Book of Rural Life, vol. 4. Chicago: Bellows-Durham, 1925.

Bowen, Louise DeKoven (Mrs. Joseph T.). "The War Work of the Women of Illinois." Paper read before the annual meeting of the Illinois Historical Society, Springfield, Illinois, May 20, 1919.

Bradley, Frances Sage, and Margaretta Williamson. *Rural Children in Selected Counties of North Carolina.* United States Children's Bureau publication no. 33. Washington: Government Printing Office, 1918.

Brainard, Annie M. *The Evolution of Public Health Nursing.* New York: W. B. Saunders, 1922. Reprint, Boston: Garland, 1985.

Breckinridge, Sophonisba. *Women in the Twentieth Century: A Study of Their Political, Social, and Economic Activities.* New York: Arno Press, 1972.

Breckinridge, Sophonisba, and Edith Abbott. "Housing Conditions in Chicago, Ill: Back of the Yards," *American Journal of Sociology* 16 (1911): 433–68.

Brown, Walter H. "Health Problems of the Foreign Born." *American Journal of Public Health* 9 (1919): 103–6.

Bunch, Mamie. "A Course for Home Demonstration Agents: The Illinois Plan." *Journal of Home Economics* 11 (1919): 431–36.

"The Care of Babies." *Illinois State Board of Health Bulletin* 6 (1910): 98.

Carpenter, Niles, and Daniel Katz. "A Study of Acculturation in the Polish Group of Buffalo, 1926–1928." *University of Buffalo Studies* 7 (1929): 101–33.

Carter, Theora. "Keep Flies Off Your Baby." *The Farmers' Wife* (May 1914): 19.

Chicago Commission on Race Relations. *The Negro in Chicago.* Chicago: University of Chicago Press, 1922.

Chicago Community Trust. *Prenatal Care in Chicago: A Survey by the Chicago Community Trust.* Chicago: Chicago Community Trust, 1922.

Chicago Department of Health. *Report for 1911–1918.* Chicago, 1919.

———. *Mortality Statistics, 1912–1918.* Chicago, 1919.

"Chicago's Baby Week." *The Survey* (June 13, 1914): 296.

Dart, Helen M. *Maternity and Child Care in Selected Rural Areas of Mississippi.* United States Children's Bureau publication no. 88. Washington: Government Printing Office, 1921.

Davis, Michael M., Jr. *Immigrant Health and the Community.* New York: Harper Brothers, 1921.

Davis, Phillip, ed. *Immigration and Americanization: Selected Readings.* Boston: Ginn, 1920.

"Decision Upholds Maternity Act." *New World* (June 13, 1923).

DeLee, Joseph B. "Progress Toward Ideal Obstetrics." *Transactions of the American Association for the Study and Prevention of Infant Mortality* 6 (1915). Reprinted in *The American Midwife Debate: A Sourcebook on Its Modern Origins,* edited by Judy Barrett Litoff. New York: Greenwood Press, 1986.

"The Delusion of Federal Aid." *Chicago Tribune* (March 29, 1923).

Department of the Interior. Bureau of Education. *Proceedings, Americanization Conference.* Washington: Government Printing Office, 1919.

"Demonstrations and Better Baby Conferences." *Illinois Health News* 8 (1922): 290–91.

Directory of Local Child-Health Agencies in the United States. United States Children's Bureau publication no. 108. Washington: Government Printing Office, 1922.

"Directory of Public Health Nurses of Illinois Outside of Chicago." *Illinois Health News* 3 (1917): 228–31.

Downey, Mrs. William. "Have You a 'Better Baby' in Your Family? Come and Find
    Out." *The Farm Home* (February 1916): 7.
"Dr. Rawlings Appointed Director." *Illinois Health News* 9 (1923): 121–31.
East, C. W. *Better Baby Conference: What It Is, Why It Is, How to Organize and
    Conduct It.* Springfield: Illinois State Department of Public Health, 1923.
"Editorial." *The Survey* (April 15, 1927): 80.
"An Effective Exhibition of a Community Survey," *The American Magazine* 12 (Feb-
    ruary 1915): 95–100.
Eldridge, Seba. *Social Legislation in Illinois.* Rockford, Ill: W. M. Shimmin, 1921.
Evans, Anne M. *Women's Rural Organizations and Their Activities.* United States
    Department of Agriculture Bulletin no. 719. Washington: Government Print-
    ing Office, 1918.
"Evans, William A.," In *Who's Who in Chicago*, edited by Albert Nelson Marquis.
    Chicago: A. N. Marquis, 1926, 281.
"The Examination and Licensure of Physicians, Other Practitioners, and Mid-
    wives." *Illinois Health News* 3 (1917): 196–99.
"Exhibit Material for Baby Week." *Illinois Health News* 3 (1917): 69.
"Famous Short Poems." *Illinois Health News* 2 (1916): 196.
"Farm Tenancy in Illinois." *The Banker-Farmer* 8 (1921): 2–3.
A farm woman. "At A Farm Women's Vacation Camp." *Wallace's Farmer* (June 17,
    1927): 7.
"Farm Women Who Count Themselves Blest By Fate." *Literary Digest* 67 (1920):
    2–53.
Farnham, Eliza W. *Life in Prairie Land.* New York: Harper, 1846. Reprint, Urbana:
    University of Illinois Press, 1988.
"Federal Aid to States a Real Menace." *Illinois Medical Journal* 40 (1921): 357.
"Fifth Annual Better Babies Conference, Illinois State Fair." *Illinois Health News* 6
    (1920): 69–75.
Fifty-third General Assembly, State of Illinois. *Senate Debates.* Springfield: Illinois
    State Register, 1923.
*Final Report of the Woman's Committee, State Council of Defense of Illinois and
    Woman's Committee, Council of National Defense, Illinois Division.* Chicago,
    1919.
"First Schools to be Held May 9 and 11." *Adams County Home Bureau Bulletin* 6
    (1928): 1.
"Flora To Have Better Baby Week," *The Southern Illinois Record*, (June 8, 1916).
"The Fly Catechism." *Illinois Farmer and Farmers' Call* (July 15, 1912): 13.
Foley, Edna L. *Visiting Nurse Manual.* Chicago: National Organization for Public
    Health Nursing, 1914.
"Foreword." *Illinois Health News* 1 (1915): 1–2.
Foster, I. A., and Harriet Fulmer. "A Health Survey of White County, Illinois." *Illi-
    nois Health News* 2 (1916): 19–36.
Fox, Elizabeth. "Rural Public Health Nursing." *Rural Health: Proceedings of the*

Second National Country Life Conference. Chicago: American Country Life Association, 1919.

Frank, Henriette Greenebaum, and Amalie Hofer Jerome, eds. *Annals of the Chicago Woman's Club.* Chicago: Chicago Woman's Club, 1916.

"Fresh Air." *Illinois Farmer and Farmers' Call* (October 1, 1911): 14.

Fulmer, Harriet. "Rural Nursing Service in Cook County." *Rural Health: Proceedings of the Second National Country Life Conference.* Chicago: American Country Life Association, 1919.

"Fulmer, Harriet (Miss)." In *The Book of Chicagoans*, edited by Albert Nelson Marquis. Chicago: A. N. Marquis, 1917, p. 251.

"Government Operation Always Costly." *Illinois Medical Journal* 41 (1922): 59.

"Governor Lowden Approves of State Medical Society Resolution." *Illinois Medical Journal* 37 (June 1920): 424.

Haasis, Bessie A. "Public Health Nursing, An Agent of Americanization." *Proceedings of the Americanization Conference.* Washington: Government Printing Office, 1919, 392–407.

Hamilton, Alice. "Excessive Child-Bearing as a Factor in Infant Mortality." *Bulletin of the American Academy of Medicine* 11 (1910): 183.

———. *Exploring the Dangerous Trades.* Boston: Little, Brown, 1943.

———. "The Social Settlement and Public Health." *Charities and the Commons* 17 (1907): 1037–40.

———. "Witchcraft on West Polk Street." *American Mercury* 10 (1927): 71–75.

Hammer, Lee F. *Recreation in Springfield.* New York: Russell Sage Foundation, 1914.

Hart, Sara L. *The Pleasure Is Mine.* Chicago: Valentine-Newman, 1947.

Harvey, Ella J. "Short Cuts in Family Doctoring." *The Practical Farmer Short Cuts for Busy Farmers, Their Wives and Families.* Philadelphia: The Practical Farmer Company, 1899.

Hbrkova, Sarka B. *Bridging the Atlantic.* Los Angeles: Adolph Herman, 1920.

"Health Centers Not Needed in Illinois." *Illinois Medical Journal* 39 (1921): 262–64.

"Health Customs and Superstitions of the Immigrant Mother." *Foreign-Born: A Bulletin of International Service* (November 1921): 332–33.

Hedger, Caroline. "The Problems of the Foreign Mother." *Child Welfare Bulletin* 7 (February 1919). Peoria, Illinois.

———. "The Relation of Health to Progress." *Illinois Farmers' Institute, Department of Household Science, Yearbook 1921.* Springfield: Illinois State Journal Company, 1921.

———. "Report of the Campaign Against Summer Diarrhea, Chicago, 1909, Under the Auspices of the Department of Health and the United Charities." *Illinois Medical Journal* 18 (1910): 534–47.

———. "The Unhealthfulness of Packingtown." *World's Work* (May 1906): 7507–10.

———. "Why the Foreign Woman Does Not Put Her Child in the Hospital." *Foreign-Born: A Bulletin of International Service* (November 1921): 340–41.

"Hedger, Caroline (Miss)." In *Who's Who in Chicago*, edited by Albert Nelson Marquis, 399. Chicago: A. N. Marquis, 1926.

Herzfeld, Elsa G. "Superstitions and Customs of the Tenement-House Mother." *Charities* 14 (1905): 985.

Hoagland, H. E. "The Movement of Rural Population in Illinois." *Journal of Political Economy* 20 (1912): 913–27.

"Home and Household." *The Prairie Farmer* (October 4, 1919): 30.

"How the Counties Stood in Federal Birth Registration Test." *Illinois Health News* 9 (1923).

"Illinois Agreement of Public Health Nursing." *Illinois Health News* 6 (1920): 163–65.

Illinois Farmer's Institute, Department of Household Science. *Yearbook 1916*. Springfield, Illinois State Journal, 1916.

———. *Yearbook 1923*. Springfield: Illinois State Journal, 1923.

Illinois General Assembly. *House Bills* 2. Springfield, 1923.

———. *Journal of the Senate* (1923). Springfield, 1923.

———. *Legislative Synopsis and Digest*. Fifty-third General Assembly. Springfield, 1923.

———. *Senate Bills* 1. Springfield, 1923.

Illinois League of Women Voters. *The First Ten Years of the Illinois League of Women Voters*. Chicago, 1930.

"Illinois State Fair Notes." *Wallace's Farmer* (August 29, 1919): 1674.

Illinois State Planning Commission. *Infant Mortality in Illinois*. Chicago, 1937.

"Important Health Legislation Fails." *Illinois Health News* 7 (1921): 1.

Infant Feeding. Springfield: Illinois State Board of Health, 1905 and 1906.

"Infant Mortality and Its Relation to Woman's Employment: A Study of Massachusetts Statistics." *Report on Condition of Woman and Child Wage-Earners in the United States*. Senate Document 645. Washington: Government Printing Office, 1912.

"Infant Welfare in Moline." *Illinois Health News* 6 (1920): 124.

"In Memoriam." *Illinois Medical Journal* 89 (1941): 358–59.

"Is the Nurse Jeopardizing the Public Health Service?" *Illinois Medical Journal* 37 (1920): 129–30.

Jenison, Marguerite Edith. *The War-Time Organization of Illinois*. Springfield: Illinois State Historical Library, 1923.

———, ed. *War Documents and Addresses*. Springfield: Illinois State Historical Library, 1923.

Joint Committee of the Chicago Medical Society and Hull House. "The Midwives of Chicago." *Journal of the American Medical Association* (April 25, 1908), pp. 1346–50.

Keating, Emmet. "Infant Welfare Society Practicing Medicine." *Illinois Medical Journal* 51 (1927): 279–81.

King, Geneva Fuller. "Report of the Nurses' Committee," *Thirtieth Annual Report of the Visiting Nurse Association of Chicago* (1920).

Kingsley, Sherman C. *Steps in the Evolution of Baby Welfare Work in Chicago.* Chicago: Elizabeth McCormick Memorial Fund, 1914.

Kirkpatrick, Ellis Lore. *The Farmer's Standard of Living.* New York: Century, 1929. Reprint, New York: Arno Press, 1971.

Krasnow, Henry. "The Foreigner a Prey of Medical Quacks." *Illinois Medical Journal* 32 (1917): 342–46.

Lathrop, Julia C. "Address." In *Illinois Farmers' Institute, Department of Household Science, Yearbook 1915.* Springfield, Illinois State Journal, 1915.

Leigh, Robert D. *Federal Health Administration in the United States.* New York: Harper and Brothers, 1927.

Leonard, Thomas H. "Rural Sanitation." In *Illinois Farmers' Institute, Department of Household Science, Yearbook 1923.* Springfield: Illinois State Journal, 1923.

"Let Us Counsel Together." *The Farmer's Wife* (September 1915): 78.

"Letters from Our Farm Women." *The Farmers' Wife* (August 1929): 12.

Loomis, Frank D. *Americanization in Chicago.* Chicago: Chicago Community Trust, 1919.

Lynd, Robert S., and Helen Merrell Lynd, *Middletown: A Study in Contemporary Culture.* New York: Harcourt Brace, 1929.

"Maternity Resolution is Paternalistic and Socialistic." *Illinois Medical Journal* 39 (1921): 375.

McAdam, George. "The National Menace of Rural Bad Health." *Outlook* (February 21, 1917): 321–27.

McDowell, Mary. "Mothers and Night Work." *The Survey* (December 22, 1917): 335.

Meigs, Grace L. "Infant Welfare Work in Wartime." *American Journal of Diseases of Children* 14 (1917): 80–97.

———. "Rural Obstetrics." *Transactions of the Seventh Annual Meeting of the American Association for Study and Prevention of Infant Mortality.* Baltimore: Franklin, 1917.

Mills, Charles F. "Proud of Your Baby?" *The Farm Home* (March 1915): 18.

Mitchell, George T. *Dr. George: An Account of the Life of a Country Doctor.* Carbondale: Southern Illinois University Press, 1994.

Moore, Elizabeth. *Maternity and Infant Care in a Rural County in Kansas.* United States Children's Bureau publication no. 26. Washington: Government Printing Office, 1917.

Mott, Frederick D., and Milton I. Roemer, *Rural Health and Medical Care.* New York: McGraw Hill, 1948.

"Mrs. H. Dunlap Started It All." *Champaign-Urbana Courier* (April 21, 1968): A-12–A-13.

National Child Welfare Association. *The American Citizen.* New York: National Child Welfare Association, n.d.

"National Maternity Bill." *The Farmer's Wife* (June 1920): 1.

Nauss, Ralph W. "Health Activities in Rural Illinois." *Illinois Health News* 9 (1923): 121–31.

———. "Typhoid Fever in Illinois." *Illinois Health News* 9 (1923): 143.

"New Contagious Disease Cards." *Illinois Health News* 2 (1916): 196.

"The New State Department of Public Health." *Illinois Health News* 3 (1917): 83–90.

"Northern Babies Fair Best." *Illinois Health News* 13 (1927): 253–56.

"Objections to the Sheppard-Towner Bill. Remarks in Opposition to Same Before the House of Representatives." *Illinois Medical Journal* 40 (1921): 143.

Olmsted, Katherine M. "Problems of Infant and Maternal Welfare Work in Rural Communities." In American Association for the Study and Prevention of Infant Mortality, *Transactions of the Ninth Annual Meeting*. Baltimore: Franklin Printing, 1919.

Our Babies: How to Keep Them Well and Happy. Springfield: Illinois State Department of Public Health, 1923.

Paradise, Viola. *Maternity and the Welfare of Young Children in a Homesteading County in Montana*. United States Children's Bureau publication no. 34. Washington: Government Printing Office, 1919.

Pehotsky, Bessie Olga. *The Slavic Immigrant Woman*. Cincinnati: Powell and White, 1925.

"Problems of the Smaller Illinois Community." *Illinois Health News* 6 (1916): 115.

"Publications of the State Board of Health." *Illinois State Board of Health Bulletin* 2 (1906): 37.

Rawlings, Isaac D. "Adequate Provision for Public Health." *Illinois Medical Journal* 9 (1923): 143–47.

———. *The Rise and Fall of Disease in Illinois*. Springfield: Illinois State Department of Public Health, 1927.

"Reject Humiliating Federal Aid." *Chicago Daily News* (March 29, 1923).

Report of the Health Insurance Commission of the State of Illinois. Springfield,1919.

"Responsibility of Mothers." *Illinois Farmer and Farmers' Call* (January 15, 1912):22.

"Reviving County Fair." *Prairie Farmer* (October 4, 1919): 34.

Ruediger, Gustav F. "A Program of Public Health for Towns, Villages, and Rural Communities." *American Journal of Public Health* 7 (1917): 235–47.

Russell Sage Foundation. *The Springfield Survey: A Study of Social Conditions in an American City*. Vol. 3. New York: Russell Sage Foundation, 1920.

"The Russian Maternity System has Destroyed, Morally as Well as Physically, a Whole Russian Generation." *Illinois Medical Journal* 43 (1923): 6.

"School Nurses Assume the Functions of Physicians." *Illinois Medical Journal* 20 (1911).

"The Senate Vote on the Sheppard-Towner Cooperation Bill." *Illinois Medical Journal* 43 (1923): 409–10.

"The Seventh Annual Better Babies Conference." *Illinois Health News* 8 (1922):291.

Seventh Annual Report of the Chief, Children's Bureau. Washington: Government Printing Office, 1919.

Shepler, Ida M. "Are Farmers' Wives Neglected and Abused?" *The Twentieth Century Farmer* (April 11, 1914).

"The Sheppard-Towner Bill as Amended is as Bad as the Original Bill." *Illinois Medical Journal* 42 (1921): 471–72.

Sherbon, Florence Brown, and Elizabeth Moore. *Maternity and Infant Care in Two Rural Counties in Wisconsin*. United States Children's Bureau publication no. 46. Washington: Government Printing Office, 1919.

"Should the Whole Family Be Eligible Under Mothers' Pension Laws?" *Illinois Medical Journal* 43 (1923): 265.

Simkhovitch, Mary Kingsbury. *The City Worker's World in America*. New York: Macmillan, 1917.

Sixth Annual Report of the Chief, Children's Bureau. Washington: Government Printing Office, 1918.

Smith, Clarence Beaman, and Meredith Chester Wilson. *The Agricultural Extension System of the United States*. New York: John Wiley and Sons, 1930.

"Some Solid Reasons for a Strike of Farm-Wives." *Literary Digest* 63 (1919): 74–78.

Sommers, Herbert J. "Infant Mortality in Rural and Urban Areas." *Public Health Service Reports* 57 (1942): 1494–1501.

"The Soviet Feature of the Sheppard Maternity Bill Exceeds in Importance the Strong Medical and Social Objections." *Illinois Medical Journal* 40 (1921): 263–64.

"The State Board of Health Exhibit." *Illinois Health News* 1 (1915): 35–43.

"The State Institute." *Prairie Farmer* (March 8, 1919): 461.

Steadman, Robert F. *Public Health Organization in the Chicago Region*. Chicago: University of Chicago Press, 1930.

Streeter, Carroll P. "What? Farm Children Healthier Than Ours?" *The Farmer's Wife* (September 1927): 519–20.

———. "Where's the Doctor When You Need Him?" *The Farmer's Wife* (December 1928).

"Summary of Child Hygiene Activities." *Illinois Health News* 9 (1923): 175.

Tilton, Fannie G. "The Value of the Country Club to the Country Woman." *Illinois Farmer and Farmers' Call* (August 1, 1911): 13.

"Typhoid Fever at Tuscola." *Illinois Health News* 2 (1916): 143.

United States Bureau of the Census. *Thirteenth Census of the United States* 4. Washington: Government Printing Office, 1914.

———. *Fourteenth Census of the United States* 6. Washington: Government Printing Office, 1923: 376–85.

———. *Fifteenth Census of the United States* 4. Washington: Government Printing Office, 1933.

————. *Sixteenth Census of the United States* 3. Washington: Government Printing Office, 1943.

United States Children's Bureau, *Directory of Local Child-Health Agencies in the United States.* Publication no. 108. Washington: Government Printing Office, 1922.

————. *The Promotion of the Welfare and Hygiene of Maternity and Infancy.* Washington: Government Printing Office, 1924.

Van Hoesen, Gertrude. "The Relation of the Home-Economics Workers to the Problems of the Foreign Woman." *Proceedings of the Americanization Conference.* Washington: Government Printing Office, 1919, 392–407.

Vincent, George E. "Better Health for Rural Communities." *Proceedings of the Second National Country Life Conference.* Chicago, 1919.

Visiting Nurse Association of Chicago, *Annual Report* (1912–1921).

Wald, Lillian D. *The House on Henry Street.* New York: Henry Holt, 1915.

Ward, Estelle Frances. "Practical Patriotism: The Work of the Woman's Defense Committee of the Council of National Defense, Illinois Division." *The Survey* (August 17, 1918): 556–58.

Ward, Florence. *The Farm Woman's Problems.* Washington: Government Printing Office, 1920.

Warner, Phoebe V. (Mrs.). "What's the Farm Woman Worth?" *The Banker-Farmer* 6 (September 1919): 12.

Webb, Ella S. "Good Health: Why Country Babies Are Not Well Developed." *The Farmers' Wife* (December 1914): 213.

"A Welcome to Women in Public Health Work." *American Journal of Public Health* 8 (February 1918): 164.

West, Mrs. Max. *Infant Care.* U.S. Children's Bureau Publication No. 8. Washington: Government Printing Office, 1914.

Whalen, Charles J. "The Abuse of Medical Charities in Chicago." *Illinois Medical Journal* 15 (1909): 1–7.

"What We Ourselves Want." *The Farmers' Wife* (September 1914): 100.

"Who Is Responsible for the Sheppard-Towner Maternity Bill?" *Illinois Medical Journal* 40 (1921): 414–15.

"Why Illinois Should Not Cooperate with the Sheppard-Towner Act." *Illinois Medical Journal* 43 (1923): 176.

"Why Young Women Are Leaving Our Farms." *Literary Digest* 67 (1920): 56–57.

Wilson, M. C., W. H. Smith, and Kathryn Van Aken Burns, *Measuring the Progress of Extension Work.* Cooperative Extension Service circular no. 104. Urbana: University of Illinois, 1929.

"Without Proof." *Illinois Health News* 2 (1916): back cover illustration.

Woman's City Club Bulletin 3–9 (1915–1921). Chicago.

"Wood, Alice Holabird (Mrs. Ira Couch Wood)," In *The Book of Chicagoans*, edited by Albert Nelson Marquis. Chicago: A. N. Marquis, 1917, 741.

Woodbury, Robert Morse. *Statures and Weights of Children Under Six Years of Age.*

United States Children's Bureau publication no. 87. Washington: Government Printing Office, 1921.

"A Worthy Exhibit." *Woman's City Club Bulletin* 3 (1915): 2.

Wright, Helen Russell. *Children of Wage-Earning Mothers: A Study of a Selected Group in Chicago.* United States Children's Bureau publication no. 102. Washington: Government Printing Office, 1922.

Secondary Sources

Adams, Jane. *The Transformation of Rural Life: Southern Illinois, 1890–1990.* Chapel Hill: University of North Carolina Press, 1994.

Antler, Joyce, and Daniel M. Fox. "The Movement Toward a Safe Maternity: Physician Accountability in New York City, 1915–1940." In *Sickness and Health in America,* edited by Judith Walzer Leavitt and Ronald L. Numbers. Madison: University of Wisconsin Press, 1985.

Apple, Rima D. *Mothers and Medicine: A Social History of Infant Feeding, 1880–1950.* Madison: University of Wisconsin Press, 1987.

———. *Vitamania: Vitamins in American Culture.* New Brunswick, N.J.: Rutgers University Press, 1996.

Bane, Juliet Lita. *The Story of Isabel Bevier.* Peoria, Ill.: Charles A. Bennett,1955.

Barrett, James R. "Americanization from the Bottom Up: Immigration and the Remaking of the Working Class in the United States, 1880–1930." *Journal of American History* 79 (1992): 996–1020.

———. *Work and Community in the Jungle.* Urbana: University of Illinois Press, 1987.

Beardsley, Edward H. "Race as a Factor in Health." In *Women, Health, and Medicine in America,* edited by Rima D. Apple. New Brunswick: Rutgers University Press, 1992.

Bellingham, Bruce, and Mary Pugh Mathis. "Race, Citizenship and Bio-politics of the Maternalist Welfare State: 'Traditional' Midwifery in the American South Under the Sheppard-Towner Act." *Social Politics* 1 (1994): 157–80.

Bennett, Michael T. "The Movement for Compulsory Health Insurance in Illinois, 1912–1920." *Illinois Historical Journal* 89 (Winter 1996): 233–46.

Blee, Kathleen M. *Women of the Klan: Racism and Gender in the 1920s.* Berkeley: University of California Press, 1991.

Bonner, Thomas Neville. *Medicine in Chicago, 1850–1950.* Urbana: University of Illinois Press, 1991.

Bowers, William L. *The Country Life Movement in America, 1900–1920.* Port Washington, N.Y.: Kennikat Press, 1974.

Bremner, Robert H., ed. *Children and Youth in America: A Documentary History.* Cambridge: Harvard University Press, 1971.

Brumberg, Joan Jacobs. *Fasting Girls: The History of Anorexia Nervosa.* New York: Plume Books, 1988.

Buechler, Steven M. *The Transformation of the Women's Suffrage Movement:*

The Case of Illinois, 1850–1920. New Brunswick: Rutgers University Press, 1986.

Buhler-Wilkerson, Karen. *False Dawn: The Rise and Decline of Public Health Nursing, 1900–1930.* New York: Garland, 1989.

Burgess, Wendy Kent. "This Beautiful Charity: Evolution of the Visiting Nurse Association of Chicago, 1889–1920." Ph.D. diss., University of Wisconsin-Milwaukee, 1990.

Burnham, John C. "Change in the Popularization of Health in the United States." *Bulletin of the History of Medicine* 58 (1984): 183–97.

Burrow, James G. *Organized Medicine in the Progressive Era: The Move Toward Monopoly.* Baltimore: Johns Hopkins University Press, 1977.

Caldwell, Mark. *The Last Crusade: The War on Consumption, 1862–1954.* New York: Atheneum, 1988.

Carlson, Robert A. "Americanization as an Early Twentieth Century Adult Education Movement." In *Americanization, Social Control, and Philanthropy,* edited by George E. Pozetta. New York: Gould, 1991.

Carlson, Shirley J. "Black Migration to Pulaski County, Illinois 1860–1900." *Illinois Historical Journal* 80 (1987): 37–47.

Carson, Mina. *Settlement Folk: Social Thought and the American Settlement Movement, 1885–1930.* Chicago: University of Chicago Press, 1990.

Castro, Felipe G., Pauline Furth, and Herbert Karlow. "The Health Beliefs of Mexican, Mexican American and Anglo American Women." *Hispanic Journal of Behavioral Sciences* 6 (1984): 365–83.

Cayleff, Susan. "Self-Help and the Patent Medicine Business." In *Women, Health, and Medicine in America,* edited by Rima D. Apple. New Brunswick, N.J.: Rutgers University Press, 1992.

Chepaitis, Joseph Benedict. "The First Federal Social Welfare Measure: The Sheppard-Towner Maternity and Infancy Act, 1918–1932." Ph.D. diss., Georgetown University, 1968.

Chesler, Ellen. *Woman of Valor: Margaret Sanger and the Birth Control Movement in America.* New York: Simon and Schuster, 1992.

Clayton, John. *The Illinois Fact Book and Historical Almanac, 1673–1968.* Carbondale: Southern Illinois University Press, 1970.

Cohen, Lizabeth. *Making a New Deal: Industrial Workers in Chicago, 1919–1939.* Cambridge, England: Cambridge University Press, 1990.

"Committee on Child Welfare," *Woman's City Club Bulletin* vol. 9, no. 11 (March 1921): 18.

Costin, Lela B. *Two Sisters for Social Justice: A Biography of Grace and Edith Abbott.* Urbana: University of Illinois Press, 1983.

Cowan, Neil M., and Ruth Schwartz Cowan. *Our Parents' Lives: The Americanization of Eastern European Jews.* New York: Basic Books, 1989.

Cowan, Ruth Schwartz. *More Work for Mother: The Ironies of Household Technology, from the Open Hearth to the Microwave.* New York: Basic Books, 1983.

Crocker, Ruth Hutchinson. *Social Work and Social Order*. Urbana: University of Illinois Press, 1992.

Cudahy, Jean M. "Report of Nurses Committee for 1918," *Twenty-ninth Annual Report of the Visiting Nurse Association of Chicago*, 12–15.

Danbom, David B. *The Resisted Revolution: Urban America and the Industrialization of Agriculture, 1900–1930*. Ames: Iowa State University Press, 1979.

———. "Romantic Agrarianism in Twentieth-Century America." *Agricultural History* 65 (1991): 1–12.

Davenport, F. Garvin. "The Sanitation Revolution in Illinois, 1870–1900." *Journal of the Illinois State Historical Society* 46 (1973): 306–26.

Davis, Allen F. *Spearheads for Reform: The Social Settlements and the Progressive Movement, 1890–1914*. New York: Oxford University Press, 1967.

Declercq, Eugene R. "The Nature and Style of Practice of Immigrant Midwives in Early Twentieth Century Massachusetts." *Journal of Social History* 19 (1985): 113–29.

DeVries, Raymond G. *Regulating Birth: Midwives, Medicine and the Law*. Philadelphia: Temple University Press, 1985.

Dolan, Jay P. *The American Catholic Experience: A History from Colonial Times to the Present*. Garden City, N.J.: Doubleday, 1985.

Drachman, Virginia G. "Female Solidarity and Professional Success: The Dilemma of Women Doctors in Late Nineteenth-Century America." *Journal of Social History* 15 (Summer 1982): 607–19.

Duffy, John. *The Sanitarians: A History of American Public Health*. Urbana: University of Illinois Press, 1990.

Dulles, Foster Rhea. *The American Red Cross: A History*. New York: Harper and Brothers, 1950.

Dwork, Deborah. *War Is Good for Babies and Other Young Children*. London: Tavistock, 1987.

Dye, Nancy Schrom. "Modern Obstetrics and Working-Class Women: The New York Midwifery Dispensary, 1890–1920." *Journal of Social History* 20 (1987): 549–64.

Esposito, Margaret. *Places of Pride: The Work and Photography of Clara R. Brian*. Bloomington, Ill.: McLean County Historical Society, 1989.

Ettling, John. *The Germ of Laziness: Rockefeller Philanthropy and Public Health in the New South*. Cambridge: Harvard University Press, 1981.

Ewen, Elizabeth. *Immigrant Women in the Land of Dollars: Life and Culture on the Lower East Side, 1890–1925*. New York: Monthly Review Press, 1985.

Ewen, Stuart. *Captains of Consciousness: Advertising and the Social Roots of the Consumer Culture*. New York: McGraw Hill, 1976.

Ewen, Stuart, and Elizabeth Ewen. *Channels of Desire*. New York: McGraw Hill, 1982.

Eyles, John, and Kevin J. Woods. *The Social Geography of Medicine and Health*. New York: St. Martin's 1983.

Fee, Elizabeth. *Disease and Discovery: A History of the Johns Hopkins School of Hygiene and Public Health.* Baltimore: Johns Hopkins University Press, 1987.

Fee, Elizabeth, and Barbara Greene. "Science and Social Reform: Women in Public Health." *Journal of Public Health Policy* 10 (1989): 161–77.

Fink, Deborah. *Agrarian Women: Wives and Mothers in Rural Nebraska, 1880–1940.* Chapel Hill: University of North Carolina Press, 1992.

Fitzpatrick, Ellen. *Endless Crusade: Women Social Scientists and Progressive Reform.* New York: Oxford University Press, 1990.

Flanagan, Maureen. "Exercising New Rights: Chicago Women's Search for Political Power Before and After Suffrage." *Social Politics* 2 (1995).

Foucault, Michel. *The Birth of the Clinic: An Archaeology of Medical Perception* translated by A. M. Sheridan Smith. New York: Pantheon, 1973.

Fox, Daniel M. *Health Policies, Health Politics: The British and American Experience, 1911–1965.* Princeton: Princeton University Press, 1986.

Fraser, Nancy. "Struggle Over Needs: Outline of a Socialist-Feminist Critical Theory of Late-Capitalist Political Culture." In *Women, the State and Welfare,* edited by Linda Gordon. Madison: University of Wisconsin Press, 1990.

Gabaccia, Donna. *From the Other Side: Women, Gender, and Immigrant Life in the U.S., 1820–1990.* Bloomington: Indiana University Press, 1994.

Garcia, Jo, Robert Kilpatrick, and Martin Richards, eds. *The Politics of Maternity Care.* Oxford: Clarendon, 1990.

Gates, Paul Wallace. *The Illinois Central Railroad and Its Colonization Work.* Cambridge: Harvard University Press, 1934.

Gear, Josephine. "The Baby's Picture: Woman as Image Maker in Small-Town America." *Feminist Studies* 13 (1987): 419–42.

Gittens, Joan. *Poor Relations: The Children of the State in Illinois, 1818–1990.* Urbana: University of Illinois Press, 1994.

Gomery, Douglas. *Shared Pleasures.* Madison: University of Wisconsin Press, 1992.

Gordon, Linda. *Heroes of Their Own Lives: The Politics and History of Family Violence.* New York: Viking Penguin, 1988.

———. *Pitied But Not Entitled: Single Mothers and the History of Welfare, 1890–1935.* New York: Free Press, 1994.

———. *Woman's Body, Woman's Right: A Social History of Birth Control in America.* New York: Viking, 1976.

———, ed. *Women, the State, and Welfare.* Madison: University of Wisconsin Press, 1990.

Graham, Otis L., Jr. *The Great Campaigns: Reform and War in America, 1900–1928.* New York: Prentice-Hall, 1971.

Green, Harvey. *The Uncertainty of Everyday Life, 1915–1945.* New York: Harper Collins, 1992.

Grey, Michael R. "Poverty, Politics, and Health: The Farm Security Administration Medical Care Program, 1935–1945." *History of Medicine and the Allied Sciences* 44 (1989): 320–50.

Haas, Shirley. *152 Years of Municipal Health Care in the City of Chicago.* Chicago: Department of Health, ca. 1980.

Hand, Wayland, ed. *American Folk Medicine: A Symposium.* Berkeley: University of California Press, 1976.

Harwood, Alan, ed. *Ethnicity and Medical Care.* Cambridge: Harvard University Press, 1981.

Hawley, Ellis W. *The Great War and the Search for a Modern Order: A History of the American People and Their Institutions.* New York: St. Martin's, 1979.

Hayden, Dolores. *The Grand Domestic Revolution: A History of Feminist Designs for American Homes, Neighborhoods, and Cities.* Cambridge: MIT Press, 1981.

Hays, Robert G., ed. *Early Stories From the Land: Short-Story Fiction from American Rural Magazines.* Urbana: University of Illinois Press, 1995.

Helman, Cecil G. *Culture. Health and Illness.* London: Wright, 1990.

Hine, Darlene Clark. *Black Women in White: Racial Conflict and Cooperation in the Nursing Profession, 1890–1950.* Bloomington: Indiana University Press, 1989.

———. "'We Specialize in the Wholly Impossible': The Philanthropic Work of Black Women." In *Lady Bountiful Revisited: Women, Philanthropy, and Power,* edited by Kathleen D. McCarthy, 70–93. New Brunswick: Rutgers University Press, 1990.

Hoffert, Sylvia D. *Private Matters: American Attitudes Toward Childbearing and Infant Nurture in the Urban North, 1800–1860.* Urbana: University of Illinois Press, 1989.

Hogan, David John. *Class and Reform: School and Society in Chicago, 1880–1930.* Philadelphia: University of Pennsylvania Press, 1985.

Holt, Marilyn Irvin. *Linoleum, Better Babies, and the Modern Farm Woman, 1890–1930.* Albuquerque: University of New Mexico Press, 1996.

Hostetler, John A. "Folk Medicine and Sympathy Healing Among the Amish." In *American Folk Medicine: A Symposium,* edited by Wayland D. Hand, 249–58. Berkeley: University of California Press, 1976.

Hoy, Suellen. *Chasing Dirt: The American Pursuit of Cleanliness.* New York: Oxford University Press, 1995.

Jellison, Katherine. *Entitled to Power: Farm Women and Technology, 1913–1963.* Chapel Hill: University of North Carolina Press, 1993.

Jensen, Joan. *Promise to the Land: Essays on Rural Women.* Albuquerque: University of New Mexico Press, 1991.

Jones, Jacquelyn. *The Dispossessed: America's Underclass from the Civil War to the Present.* New York: Basic Books, 1992.

Jurczak, Charles Andrew. "Ethnicity, Status, and Generational Positioning: A Study of Health Practices Among Polonians in Five Ethnic Islands." Ph.D. diss., University of Pittsburgh, 1964.

Kauffman, Christopher J. *Ministry and Meaning: A Religious History of Catholic Health Care in the United States.* New York: Crossroad, 1995.

Kennedy, David M. *Birth Control in America: The Career of Margaret Sanger.* New Haven: Yale University Press, 1970.

———. *Over Here: The First World War and American Society.* Oxford: Oxford University Press, 1980.

Kirschner, Don S. *City and Country: Rural Responses to Urbanization in the 1920s.* Westport, Conn.: Greenwood, 1970.

Klaus, Alisa. "Depopulation and Race Suicide: Maternalism and Pronatalist Ideologies in France and the United States." In *Mothers of a New World: Maternalist Politics and the Origins of Welfare States,* edited by Seth Koven and Sonya Michel. New York: Routledge, 1993.

———. *Every Child a Lion: The Origins of Maternal and Infant Health Policy in the United States and France, 1890–1920.* Ithaca: Cornell University Press, 1993.

———. "Women's Organizations and the Infant Health Movement in France and the United States, 1890–1920." In *Lady Bountiful Revisited: Women, Philanthropy, and Power,* edited by Kathleen D. McCarthy. New Brunswick: Rutgers University Press, 1990.

Knowles, Jane B. "'It's Our Turn Now': Rural Women Speak Out, 1900–1920." In *Women and Farming: Changing Roles, Changing Structures,* edited by Wava G. Haney and Jane B. Knowles. Boulder, Colo.: Westview Press, 1988.

Kobrin, Frances E. "The American Midwife Controversy: A Crisis in Professionalization." *Bulletin of the History of Medicine* 40 (1966): 350–63.

Koven, Seth, and Sonya Michel, eds. *Mothers of a New World: Maternalist Politics and the Origins of Welfare States.* New York: Routledge, 1993.

Krause, Corinne Azen. "Urbanization Without Breakdown: Italian, Jewish, and Slavic Immigrant Women in the United States, 1890–1891." *Journal of Urban History* (1978): 291–305.

Kraut, Alan M. *Silent Travelers: Germs, Genes and the "Immigrant Menace."* Baltimore: Johns Hopkins University Press, 1994.

Kula, Witold, Nina Assorodobraj-Kula, and Marcin Kula, eds. *Writing Home: Immigrants in Brazil and the United States, 1890–1891.* New York: Columbia University Press, 1986.

Ladd-Taylor, Molly. *Mother-Work: Women, Child Welfare, and the State, 1890–1930.* Urbana: University of Illinois Press, 1994.

———. *Raising a Baby the Government Way.* New Brunswick: Rutgers University Press, 1986.

Lears, T. J. Jackson. "From Salvation to Self-Realization: Advertising and the Therapeutic Roots of the Consumer Culture, 1880–1930." In *The Culture of Consumption: Critical Essays in American History, 1880–1980,* edited by Richard Wightman Fox and T. J. Jackson Lears. New York: Pantheon, 1983.

Leavitt, Judith Walzer. "Birthing and Anesthesia: The Debate Over Twilight Sleep." *Signs* 6 (1980): 147–64.

———. *Brought to Bed: Childbearing in America*. New York: Oxford University Press, 1986.

———. *The Healthiest City: Milwaukee and the Politics of Health Reform*. Princeton: Princeton University Press, 1982.

———. *Typhoid Mary: Captive to the Public's Health*. Boston: Beacon Press, 1996.

Lemons, J. Stanley. *The Woman Citizen: Social Feminism in the 1920s*. Urbana: University of Illinois, 1973.

Lentzner, Harold Roy. "Seasonal Patterns of Infant and Child Mortality in New York, Chicago and New Orleans, 1870–1919." Ph.D. diss., University of Pennsylvania, 1987.

Link, Arthur S. *Wilson: The Struggle for Neutrality, 1914–1915*. Princeton: Princeton University Press, 1960.

Link, Arthur S., and Richard L. McCormick, eds. *Progressivism*. Arlington Heights, Ill.: Harlan Davidson, 1983.

Lissak, Rivka Shpak. *Pluralism and Progressives: Hull House and the New Immigrants, 1890–1919*. Chicago: University of Chicago Press, 1989.

Litoff, Judy Barrett. *American Midwives, 1860 to the Present*. Westport, Conn.: Greenwood, 1978.

———, ed. *The American Midwife Debate: A Sourcebook on Its Modern Origins*. New York: Greenwood, 1986.

Loudon, Irvine. "Maternal Mortality: 1880–1950. Some Regional and International Comparisons." *Social History of Medicine* 1 (August 1988): 183–228.

Lunbeck, Elizabeth. *The Psychiatric Persuasion: Knowledge, Gender, and Power in Modern America*. Princeton: Princeton University Press, 1994.

Maloney, Clarence, ed. *The Evil Eye*. New York: Columbia University Press, 1976.

Marquis, Albert Nelson, ed. *The Book of Chicagoans*. Chicago: A. N. Marquis, 1917 and 1926.

Marti, Donald B. *Women of the Grange: Mutuality and Sisterhood in Rural America, 1866–1920*. New York: Greenwood, 1991.

May, Lary. *Screening Out the Past: The Birth of Mass Culture and the Motion Picture Industry*. New York: Oxford University Press, 1980.

McCarthy, Kathleen. *Noblesse Oblige: Charity and Cultural Philanthropy in Chicago, 1849–1929*. Chicago: University of Chicago Press, 1982.

McCarthy, Kathleen D. "Parallel Power Structures: Women and the Voluntary Sphere." In *Lady Bountiful Revisited: Women, Philanthropy, and Power*, edited by Kathleen D. McCarthy. New Brunswick: Rutgers University Press, 1990.

McClymer, John F. "Gender and the 'American Way of Life': Women in the Americanization Movement." *Journal of American Ethnic History* 10 (1991): 3–20.

———. *War and Welfare: Social Engineering in America, 1890–1925*. Westport, Conn.: Greenwood, 1980.

McKinney, Rhondal. "Clara Brian: Home Bureau Photographs, 1919–1926." Exhibition catalogue. Bloomington, Ill.: McLean County Historical Society, n.d.

Meckel, Richard A. "Judging Progressive Era Infant Welfare in Light of *Fatal Years* — and Vice Versa." *Bulletin of the History of Medicine* 68 (1994): 105–12.
———. *Save the Babies: American Public Health Reform and the Prevention of Infant Mortality, 1850–1929.* Baltimore: Johns Hopkins University Press, 1990.

Melosh, Barbara. *The Physician's Hand.* Philadelphia: Temple University Press, 1982.

Michel, Sonya, and Robyn Rosen. "The Paradox of Maternalism: Elizabeth Lowell Putnam and the American Welfare State." *Gender and History* 4 (1992): 364–86.

Miller, Katherine Aird, and Raymond H. Montgomery. *A Chautauqua to Remember: The Story of Old Salem.* Petersburg, Ill.: Silent River Press, 1987.

Morantz, Regina Markell. "Making Women Modern: Middle Class Women and Health Reform in the Nineteenth Century." In *Women and Health in America*, edited by Judith Walzer Leavitt. Madison: University of Wisconsin Press, 1994.

Muncy, Robyn. *Creating a Female Dominion in American Reform, 1890–1935.* New York: Oxford University Press, 1991.

Nelli, Humbert S. *Italians in Chicago, 1880–1920.* London: Oxford University Press, 1970.

Neth, Mary. *Preserving the Family Farm.* Baltimore: Johns Hopkins University Press, 1995.

Numbers, Ronald L. *Almost Persuaded: American Physicians and Compulsory Health Insurance, 1912–1920.* Baltimore: Johns Hopkins University Press, 1978.
———. "Do-It-Yourself the Sectarian Way." In *Medicine Without Doctors*, edited by Guenter B. Risse, Ronald L. Numbers, and Judith Walzer Leavitt, 49–72. New York: Science History Publications, 1977.
———. "The History of American Medicine: A Field in Ferment," in *The Promise of American History* ed. Stanley L. Kutler and Stanley N. Katz. Baltimore: Johns Hopkins University Press, 1982, 245–64.

Oates, Mary J. *The Catholic Philanthropic Tradition in America.* Bloomington: Indiana University Press, 1995.

Pegram, Thomas R. *Partisans and Progressives: Private Interest and Public Policy in Illinois, 1870–1922.* Urbana: University of Illinois Press, 1992.
———. "Public Health and Progressive Dairying in Illinois." *Agricultural History* 65 (1991): 36–50.

Pernick, Martin S. *The Black Stork: Eugenics and the Death of "Defective" Babies in American Medicine and Motion Pictures Since 1915.* New York: Oxford University Press, 1996.

Phillips, Anne. *Engendering Democracy.* University Park: Pennsylvania University Press, 1991.

Philpott, Thomas Lee. *The Slum and the Ghetto: Immigrants, Blacks, and Reformers in Chicago, 1880–1930.* Belmont, Calif.: Wadsworth Press, 1991.

Pill, Roisin, and Noel C. H. Stott. "Concepts of Illness Causation and Responsibility: Some Preliminary Data from a Sample of Working-Class Mothers." *Social Science and Medicine* 16 (1982): 43–52.

Piven, Frances Fox. "Ideology and the State: Women, Power, and the Welfare State." In *Women, the State and Welfare*, edited by Linda Gordon. Madison: University of Wisconsin Press, 1990.

Porter, Roy. "The Patient's View: Doing Medical History from Below." *Theory and Society* 14 (1985): 175–98.

Preston, Samuel H., and Michael R. Haines. *Fatal Years: Child Mortality in Late Nineteenth Century America*. Princeton: Princeton University Press, 1991.

Radzialowski, Thaddeus C. "'Let Us Join Hands': The Polish Women's Alliance." In *Immigrant Women*, edited by Maxine Schwartz Seller. Philadelphia: Temple University Press, 1981.

Ragucci, Antoinette T. "Generational Continuity and Change in Concepts of Health, Curing Practices, and Ritual Expressions of the Women of an Italian-American Enclave." Ph.D. diss., Boston University, 1971.

———. "Italian Americans." In *Ethnicity and Medical Care*, edited by Alan Harwood, 216–47. Cambridge: Harvard University Press, 1981.

Reagan, Leslie J. "About to Meet Her Maker: Women, Doctors, Dying Declarations, and the State's Investigation of Abortion, Chicago, 1867–1940." *Journal of American History* 77 (March 1991): 1240–64.

———. *When Abortion Was a Crime: Women, Medicine and Law in the United States, 1867–1973*. Berkeley: University of California Press, 1997.

Reilinger, Elizabeth G. "Child Health and the State: The Evolution of Federal Policy." Ph.D. diss., Cornell University, 1980.

Reverby, Susan M. *Ordered to Care: The Dilemma of American Nursing, 1850–1945*. Cambridge, England: Cambridge University Press, 1987.

Rodgers, Daniel T. "In Search of Progressivism." *Reviews in American History* 10 (1982): 113–32.

Rogers, Naomi. *Dirt and Disease: Polio Before FDR*. New Brunswick: Rutgers University Press, 1992.

———. "Dirt, Flies, and Immigrants: Explaining the Epidemiology of Poliomyelitis, 1900–1916." *Journal of the History of Medicine and Allied Sciences* 44 (1989): 486–505.

———. "Women and Sectarian Medicine." In *Women, Health, and Medicine in America*, edited by Rima D. Apple. New Brunswick: Rutgers University Press, 1992.

Rosen, George. "The First Neighborhood Health Center Movement: Its Rise and Fall." In *Sickness and Health in America*, edited by Judith Walzer Leavitt and Ronald L. Numbers. Madison: University of Wisconsin Press, 1985.

———. *Preventive Medicine in the United States, 1900–1975*. New York: Science History Publications, 1975.

Rosenberg, Charles E. "Social Class and Medical Care in 19th-Century America:

The Rise and Fall of the Dispensary." In *Sickness and Health in America*, edited by Judith Walzer Leavitt and Ronald L. Numbers. Madison: University of
Wisconsin Press, 1985.

Rosenkrantz, Barbara Gutman. *Public Health and the State: Changing Views in
Massachusetts, 1842–1936*. Cambridge: Harvard University Press, 1972.

Ross, Ellen. *Love and Toil: Motherhood in Outcast London, 1870–1918*. New York:
Oxford University Press, 1993.

Rothman, Sheila M. "Women's Clinics or Doctors' Offices?: The Sheppard-Towner
Act and the Promotion of Preventive Health Care." In *Social History and So-
cial Policy*, edited by David J. Rothman and Stanton Wheeler. New York:
Academic Press, 1981.

Sarvasy, Wendy. "Beyond the Difference versus Equality Debate: Postsuffrage Feminism, Citizenship, and the Quest for a Feminist Welfare State." *Signs* 17
(1992): 329–62.

————. "From Man and Philanthropic Service to Feminist Social Citizenship."
Social Politics 1 (1994): 306–25.

Schackel, Sandra. *Social Housekeepers: Women Shaping Public Policy in New Mexico, 1920–1940*. Albuquerque: University of New Mexico Press, 1992.

Scott, Roy V. *The Reluctant Farmer: The Rise of Agricultural Extension to 1914*.
Urbana: University of Illinois Press, 1970.

Seller, Maxine. "The Education of the Immigrant Woman, 1900–1935." *Journal of
Urban History* 4 (1978): 307–30.

Settensen, Margaret, and Larry Colker. "Intercultural Misunderstandings About
Health Care." *Social Science and Medicine* 16 (1982): 1949–54.

Shanabruch, Charles. *Chicago's Catholics*. Notre Dame, IN: University of Notre
Dame Press, 1981.

Shapiro, Laura. *Perfection Salad: Women and Cooking at the Turn of the Century*.
New York: Farrar, Straus, and Giroux, 1986.

Sklar, Kathryn Kish. *Florence Kelley and the Nation's Work*. New Haven: Yale University Press, 1995.

————. "The Historical Foundations of Women's Power in the Creation of the
American Welfare State, 1830–1930." In *Mothers of a New World: Maternalist
Politics and the Origins of Welfare States*, edited by Seth Koven and Sonya
Michel, pp. 43–93. New York: Routledge, 1993.

————. "Who Funded Hull House?" In *Lady Bountiful Revisited: Women, Philanthropy, and Power*, edited by Kathleen D. McCarthy. New Brunswick: Rutgers
University Press, 1990.

Skocpol, Theda. *Protecting Soldiers and Mothers: The Politics of Social Provision
in the United States, 1870s–1920s*. Cambridge: Harvard University Press,
1992.

Slayton, Robert A. *Back of the Yards: The Making of a Local Democracy*. Chicago:
University of Chicago Press, 1986.

Sloan, Kay. *The Loud Silents: Origins of the Social Problem Film.* Urbana: University of Illinois Press, 1988.

Smith, Susan Lynn. "'Sick and Tired of Being Sick and Tired': Black Women and the National Negro Health Movement, 1915–1950." Ph.D. diss., University of Wisconsin, 1991.

Smukstra, Michael J. "Work and Family: Farm Women in Illinois, 1820–1915." Ph.D. diss., Northern Illinois University, 1991.

Spector, Rachel E. *Cultural Diversity in Health and Illness.* New York: Appleton-Century Crofts, 1979.

Stadum, Beverly. *Poor Women and Their Families: Hard Working Charity Cases, 1900–1930.* Albany: State University of New York Press, 1992.

Starr, Paul. *The Social Transformation of American Medicine.* New York: Basic Books, 1982.

Stevens. Rosemary. *American Medicine and the Public Interest.* New Haven: Yale University Press, 1971.

———. *In Sickness and In Wealth: American Hospitals in the Twentieth Century.* New York: Basic Books, 1989.

Strasser, Susan. *Never Done: A History of American Housework.* New York: Pantheon, 1982.

Sturgis, Cynthia. "'How're You Gonna Keep 'Em Down on the Farm?'": Rural Women and the Urban Model in Utah." *Agricultural History* 60 (1986): 182–215.

Tingley, Donald F. *The Structuring of a State: The History of Illinois, 1899–1928.* Urbana: University of Illinois Press, 1980.

Tomes, Nancy. *The Gospel of Germs: Men, Women, and the Microbe in American Life.* Cambridge: Harvard University Press, 1998.

———. "The Private Side of Public Health: Sanitary Science, Domestic Hygiene, and the Germ Theory, 1870–1990." *Bulletin of the History of Medicine* 64 (1990): 509–39.

Urofsky, Melvin I., ed. *Documents of American Legal History.* New York: Knopf, 1989.

Vinikas, Vincent. *Soft Soap, Hard Sell: American Hygiene in an Age of Advertisement.* Ames: Iowa State University Press, 1992.

Waller, Gregory A. *Main Street Amusements.* Washington: Smithsonian Institution Press, 1995.

Wertz, Richard W., and Dorothy C. Wertz. *Lying-In: A History of Childbirth in America.* New York: Free Press, 1977.

Wheeler, Adade Mitchell, with Marlene Stein Wortman. *The Roads They Made: Women in Illinois History.* Chicago: Kerr, 1977.

Wiebe, Robert H. *The Search for Order, 1877–1920.* New York: Hill and Wang, 1967.

Woloch, Nancy, ed. Introduction to *Muller v. Oregon: A Brief History with Documents.* New York: St. Martin's Press, 1996.

Wynn, Neil A. *From Progressivism to Prosperity: World War I and American Society.* New York: Holmes and Meier, 1986.

Young, James Harvey. *The Medical Messiahs: A Social History of Health Quackery in Twentieth-Century America.* Princeton: Princeton University Press, 1967.

Zelizer, Viviana A. *Pricing the Priceless Child: The Changing Social Value of Children.* New York: Basic Books, 1985.

INDEX

Women and Health Series
Cultural and Social Perspectives
Rima D. Apple and Janet Golden, Editors

The series examines the social and cultural construction
of health practices and policies, focusing on women as subjects and objects
of medical theory, health services, and policy formulation.

MOTHERS AND MOTHERHOOD: *Readings in American History*
Edited by Rima D. Apple and Janet Golden

MAKING MIDWIVES LEGAL: *Childbirth, Medicine, and the Law,*
Second Edition
Raymond G. DeVries

THE SELLING OF CONTRACEPTION: *The Dalkon Shield Case,*
Sexuality, and Women's Autonomy
Nicole J. Grant

AND SIN NO MORE: *Social Policy and Unwed Mothers in Cleveland,*
1855–1990
Marian J. Morton

WOMEN AND PRENATAL TESTING: *Facing the Challenges of*
Genetic Technology
Edited by Karen H. Rothenberg and Elizabeth J. Thomson

WOMEN'S HEALTH: *Complexities and Differences*
Edited by Sheryl Burt Ruzek, Virginia L. Olesen, and Adele E. Clarke

LISTEN TO ME GOOD: *The Life Story of an Alabama Midwife*
Margaret Charles Smith and Linda Janet Holmes